THE WIT & WISDOM OF

RATAN TATA

The Wit & Wisdom of

Ratan Tata

HAY HOUSE INDIA
New Delhi • London • Sydney
Carlsbad, California • New York City

Hay House Publishers (India) Pvt Ltd
Muskaan Complex, Plot No. 3, B-2, Vasant Kunj, New Delhi – 110070, India

Hay House LLC, P.O. Box 5100, Carlsbad, CA 92018-5100, USA
Hay House UK Ltd, 1st Floor, Crawford Corner, 91-93 Baker Street, London W1U 6QQ, UK
Hay House Australia Publishing Pty Ltd, 18/36 Ralph St., Alexandria NSW 2015, Australia

Email: contact@hayhouse.co.in
Website: www.hayhouse.co.in

Images provided by the Tata Central Archives.

Designed by Raghav Khattar at Hay House India

First published by Hay House Publishers India, 2018
Reprint, 2025
20 19 18 17 16 15 14 13 12 11

ISBN 978-93-85827-29-7

Printed at Thomson Press

JAMSETJI TATA

&

J. R. D. TATA

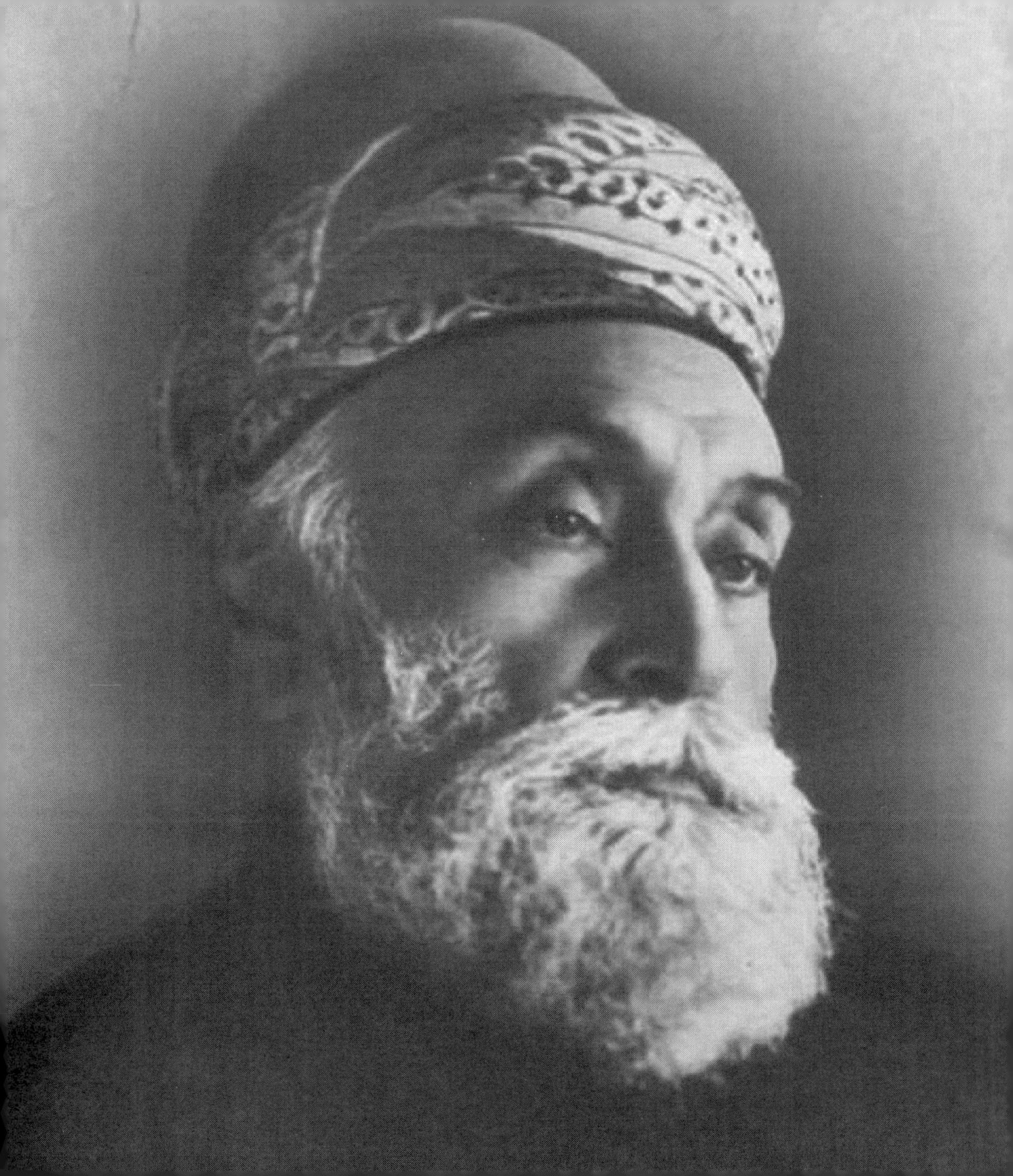

Jamsetji believed that India would have truly laid aside its imperialist yoke only when it realized the full potential of its natural resources and became a modern, industrial nation. Over a hundred years later, as India still continues on that journey, his vision remains the Group's main guiding force.

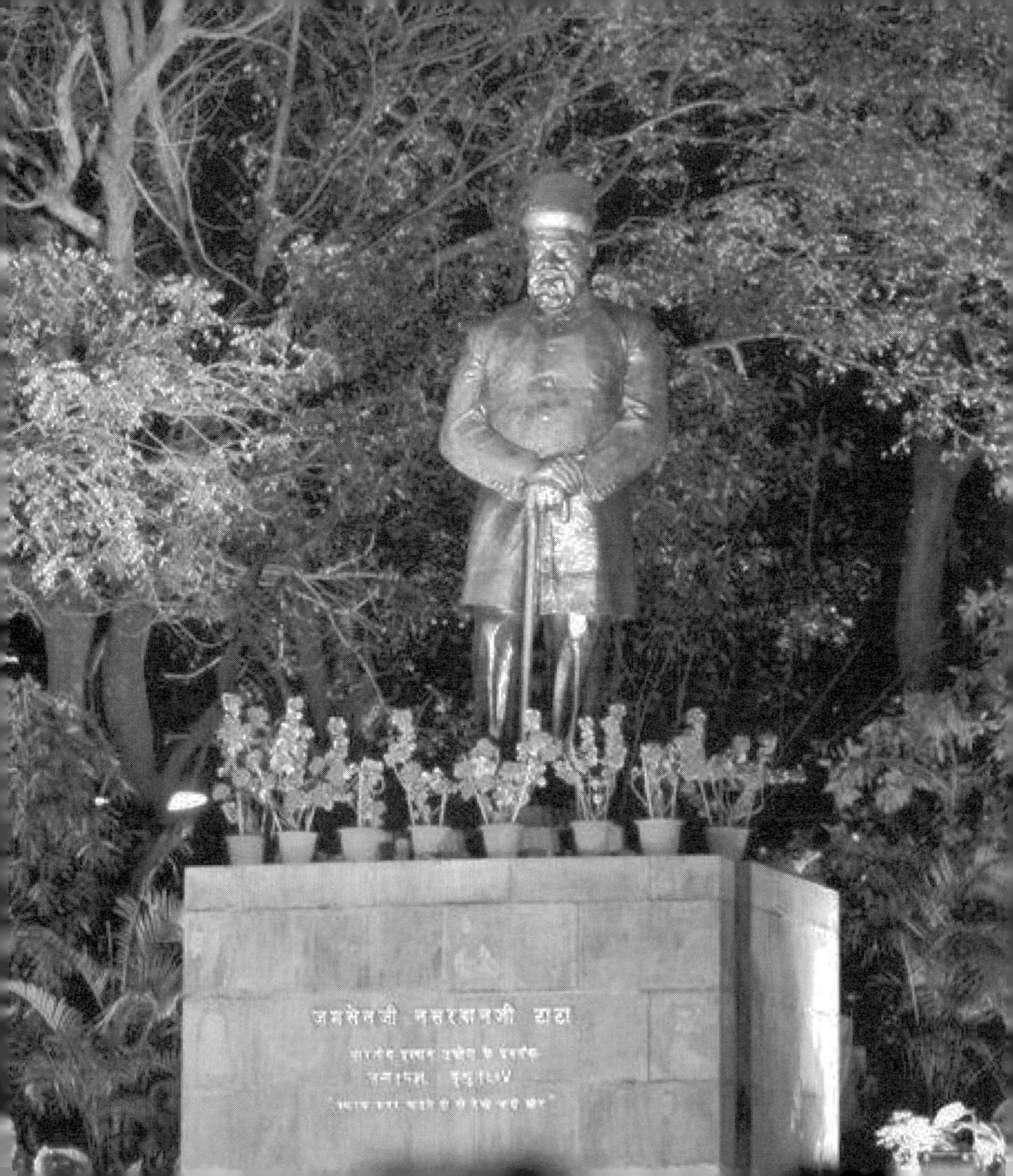

Jamsetji saw disciplines such as medicine and science and industries such as energy and steel as building blocks in the emergence of a brave and bright new country. After creating the most modern textile mills, he committed the Group to setting up India's first steel plant and the first hydroelectricity plant and bestowed half his personal wealth to found the country's first institution of higher learning, the Indian Institute of Science. Thus did he set the mandate for the Group: to look beyond the generation of products and profits to serving the communities in which Tata companies functioned.

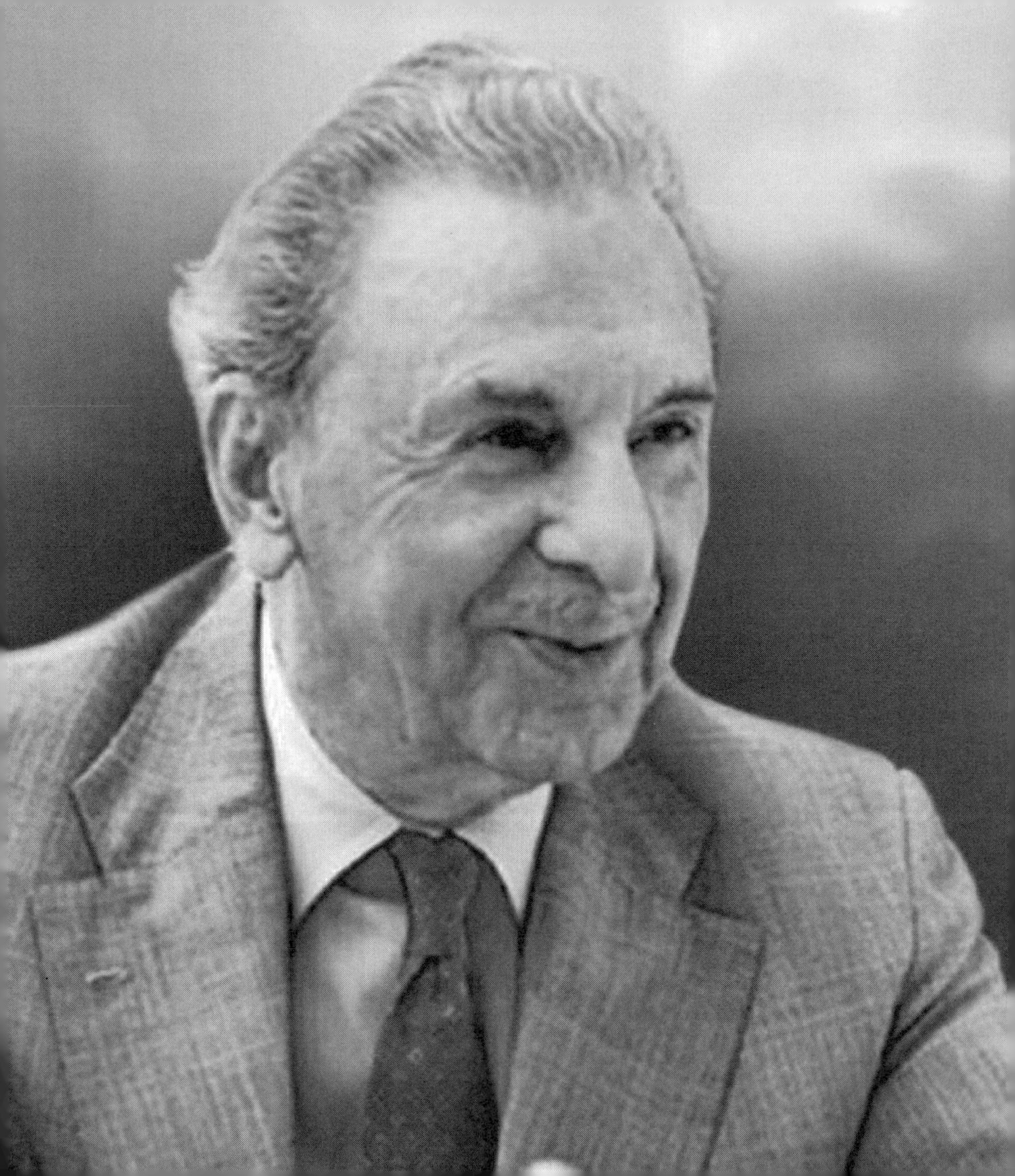

JRD's outstanding contribution, the greatest among the many he made, was to expand the group on the basis of principles and values and ethics. He worked in a world of onerous regulations. He had the courage to object to them publicly, but he never broke the law. JRD imparted the discipline that he expected his people to follow. Never, not once, did he cut corners or find a loophole. Nor did he ask anyone to do so.

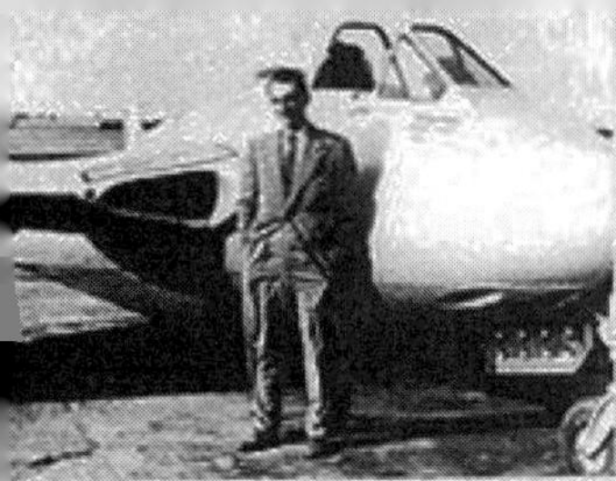

JANUARY 20 1952

...ata in front of a jet propeller "Vampire", signifying the shape of things to come for the civil aviation industry of a young India

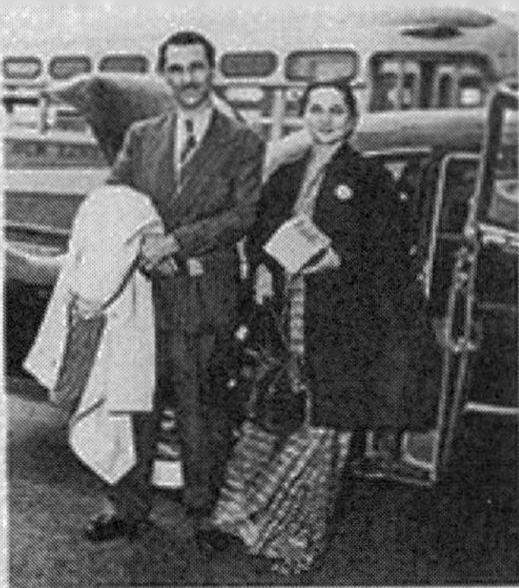

OCTOBER 20 1957

JRD Tata with wife Thelma

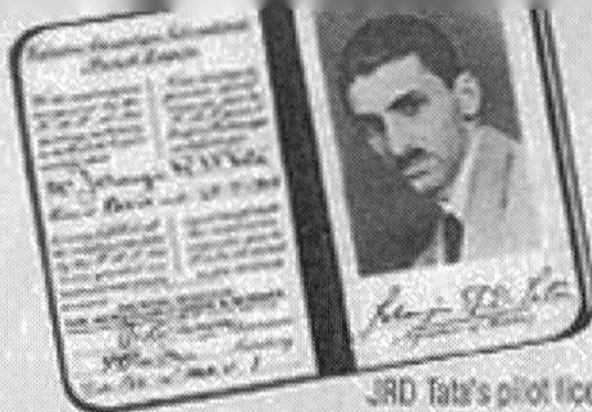

JULY 29, 1904

JRD Tata's pilot licence

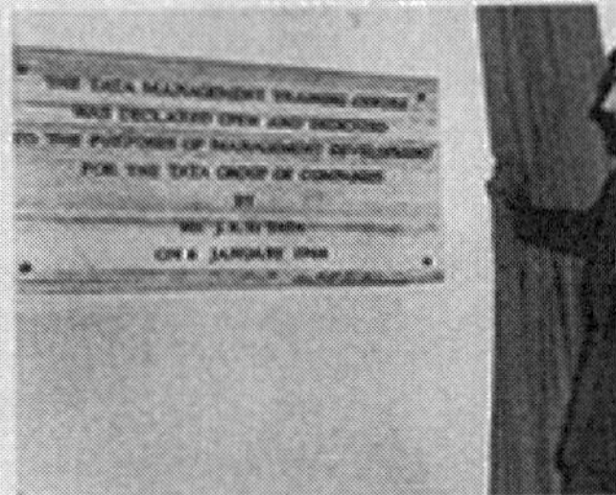

JRD Tata inaugurating the Tata Management Training Ce...

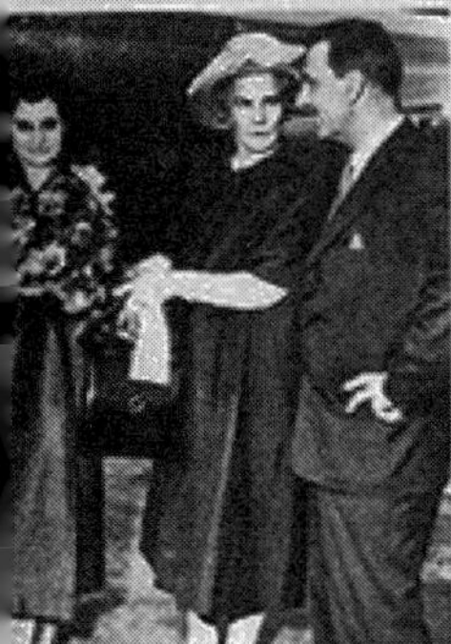

JUNE 8 1948

...D Tata at the inaugural trans-atlantic flight of Air India with Indira Gandhi

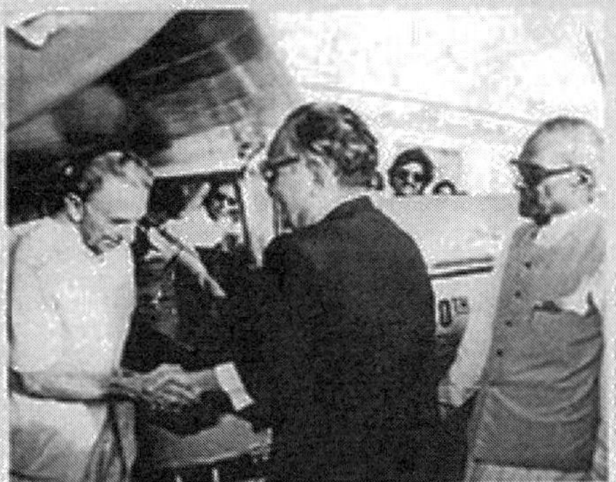

16 OCTOBER 1982

JRD Tata welcomed by MM Salim, MD, PIA when he landed at Karachi in his single-engined Leopard Moth aircraft to commemorate the 50th anniversary of his pioneering Karachi-Bombay solo flight made in 1932.

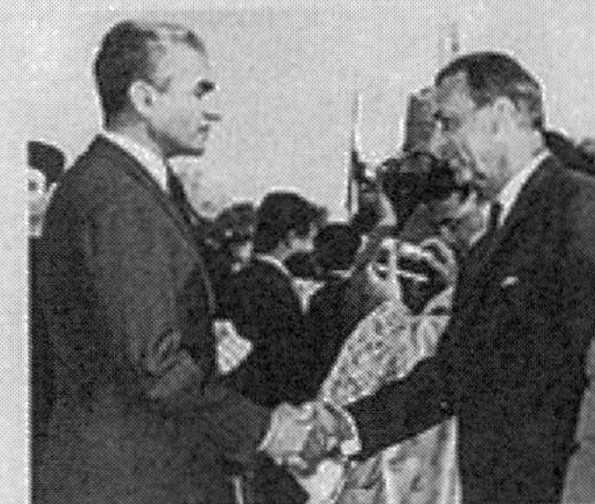

Shah of Iran's visit ...

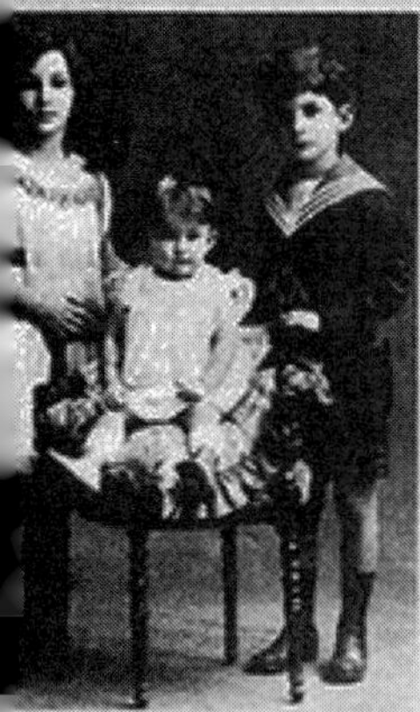

...D Tata with his brother and sister

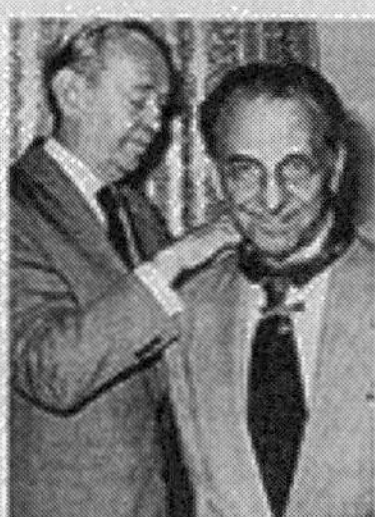

1978

J.R.D. Tata receives the Knights Commander Cross Award from the German Ambassador in Bombay

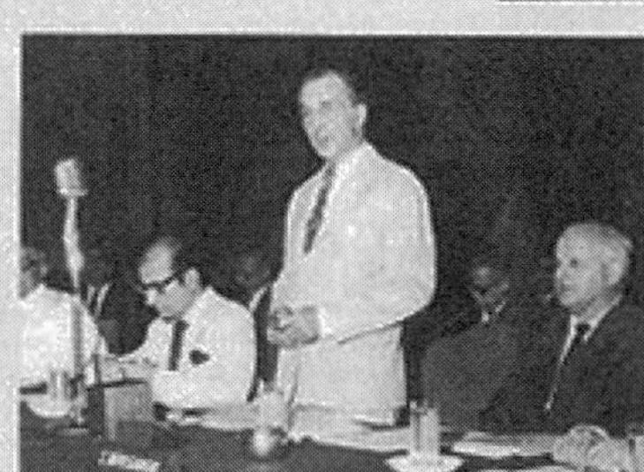

AUGUST 21, 1974

JRD Tata addressing the Annual General Meeting of TISCO in Bombay. To his right is NA Palkhivala, deputy chairman and to his left S Moolgaokar, vice chairma...

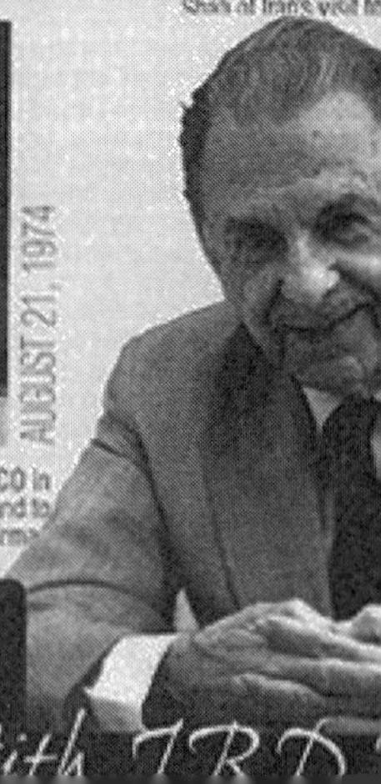

Down Memory Lane

With JRD...

VIGNETTES FROM THE LIFE AND TIMES OF BUSINESS MAHARAJAS

Business was but one facet of the JRD mosaic. He played the part of statesman in India and abroad. He espoused causes like family planning and, in his later years, became a staunch supporter of women's rights, and had deep concern for the plight of the girl child.

HIS YEARS AS

TATA GROUP CHAIRMAN

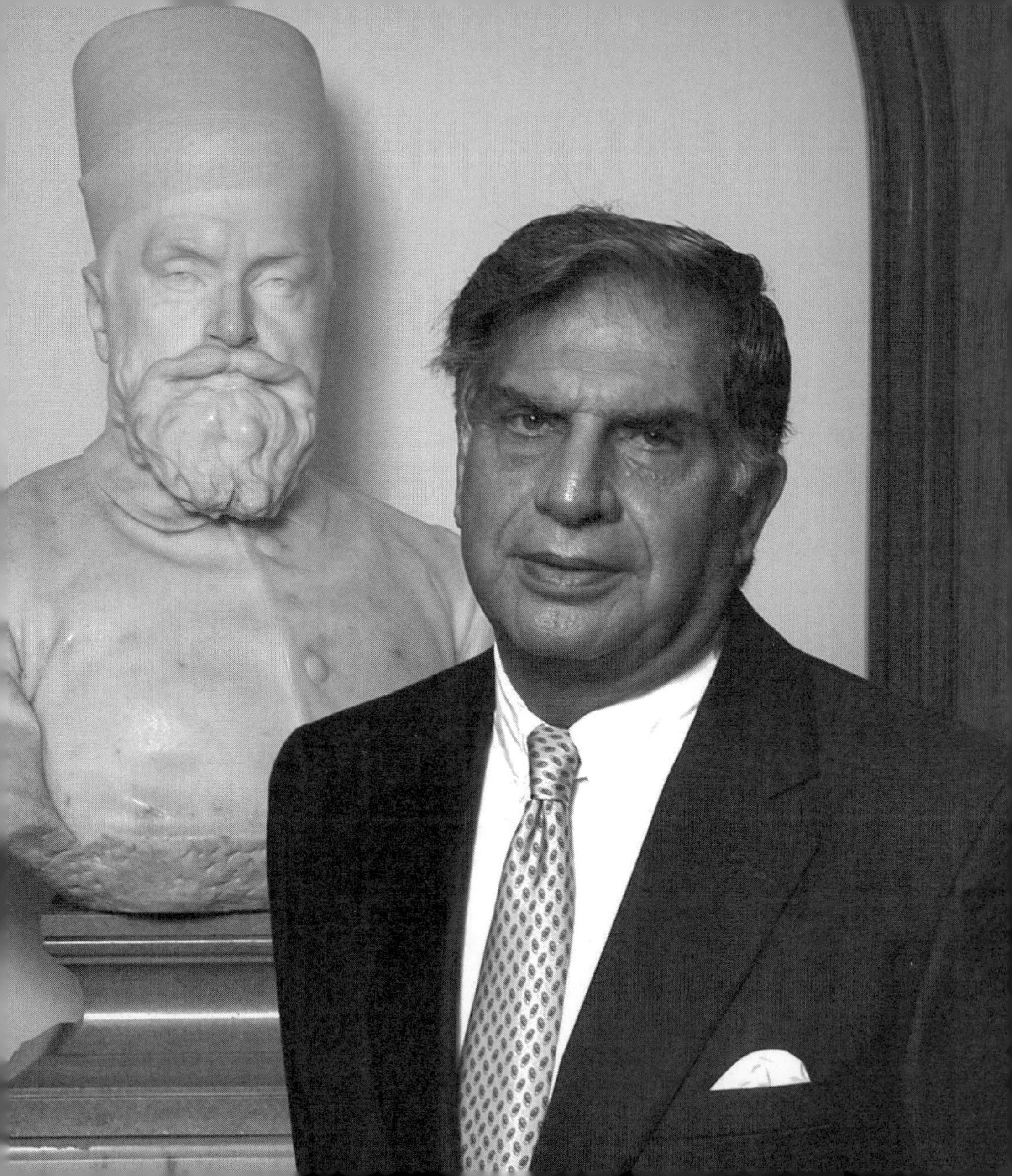

I was wearing the boots of a person who was a legend, and I asked myself, what should I do? And, I decided, the worst thing I could do was to copy him or be him, because I could never be J.R.D. Tata. So what I should do is just be myself, operate on the values that I had in me anyway, and do whatever I thought was right for the group. Similarly, I should not look for someone who is my carbon copy. That would be wrong.

(March 2002)

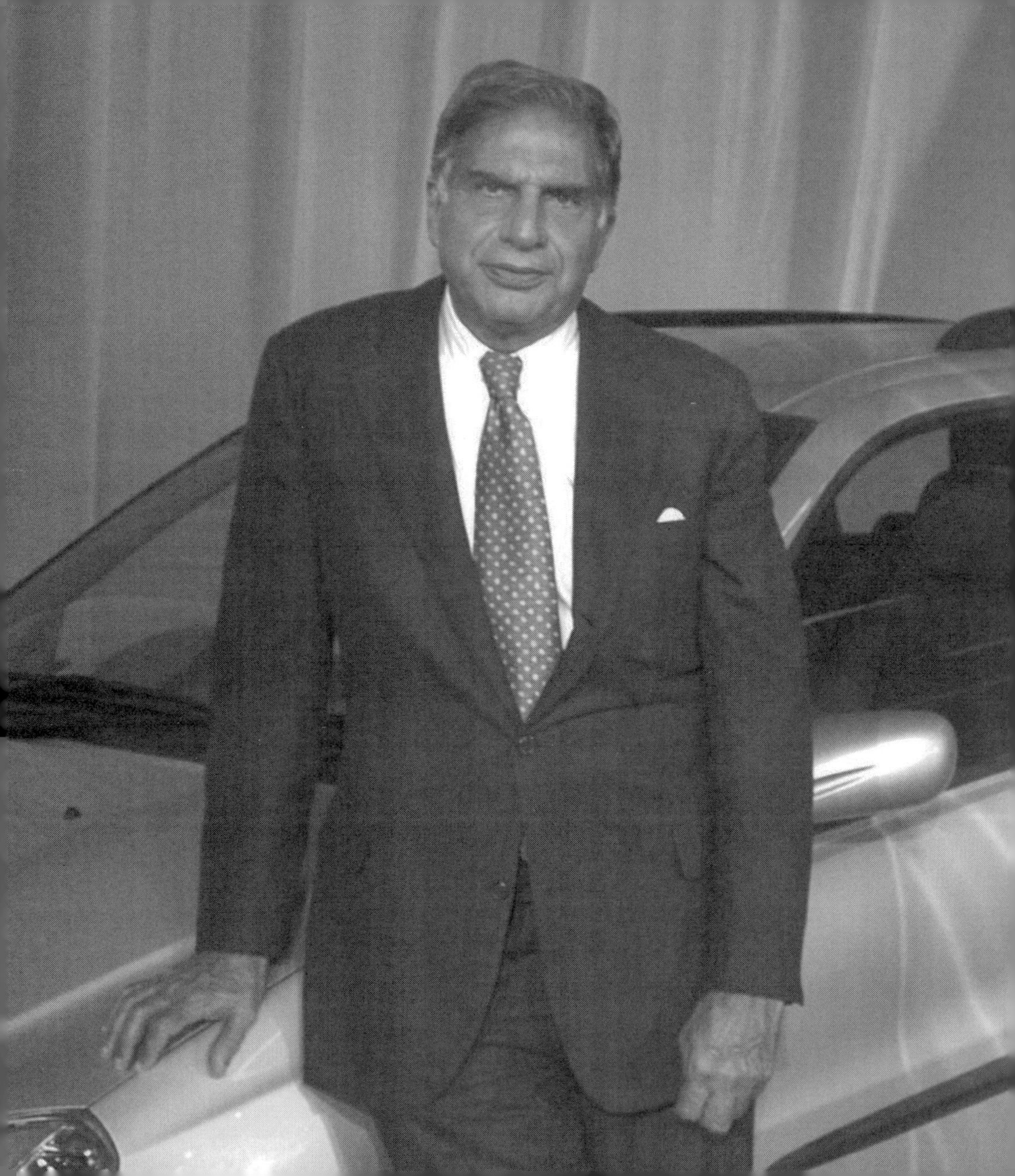

From 1962 onwards, my life has been about living in different Tata organizations in different positions. Each of these experiences has had its attributes, its pulls and pressures.

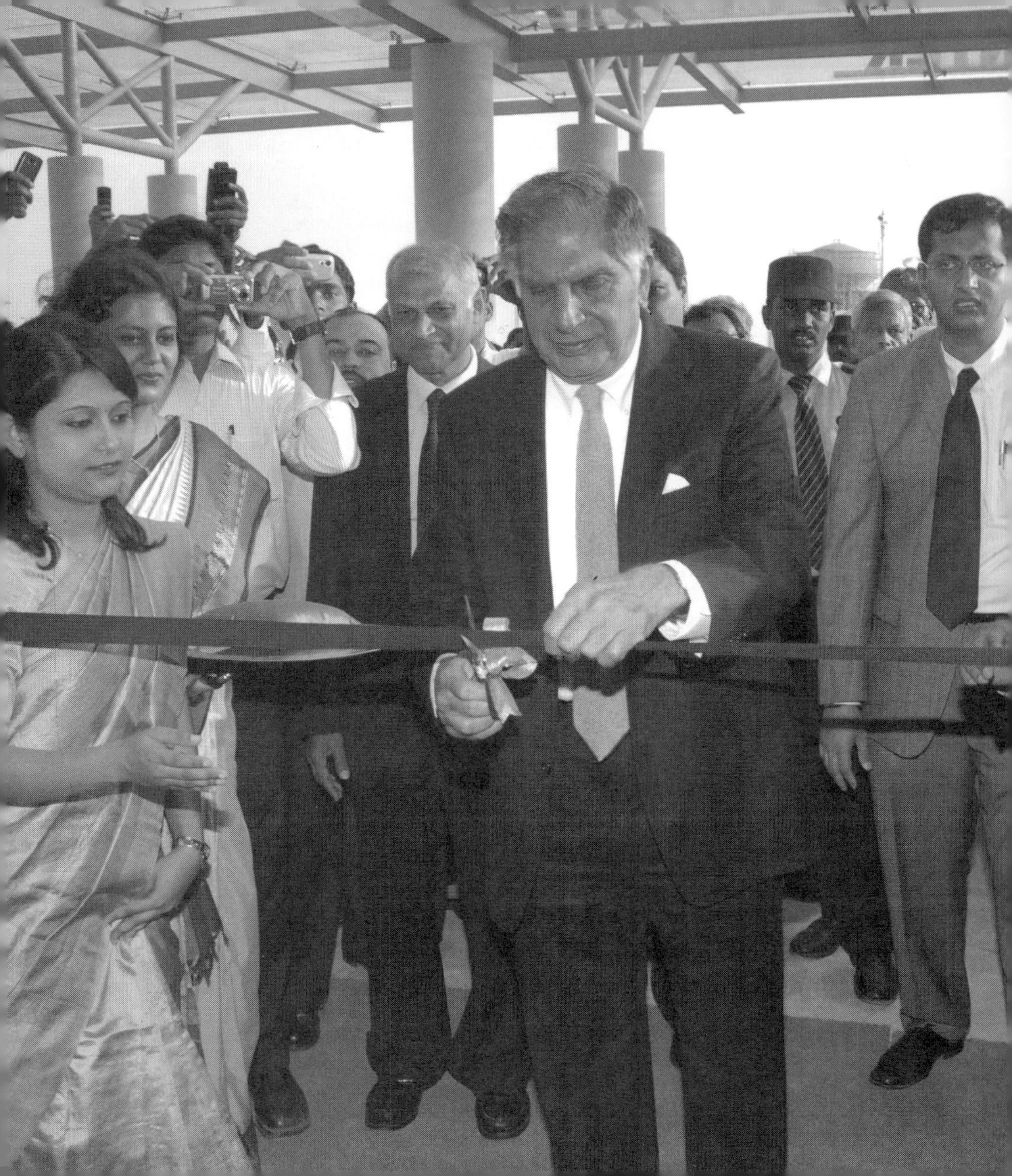

It hasn't felt like a job; it's been more like a personal issue. It hasn't been for money and it hasn't been for visibility. It's just been the challenge and, to a great extent, the passion . . .

I kept saying, please question the unquestionable. I tried to tell our younger managers, 'Don't just accept something that was done in the past, don't accept something as a holy cow. Go question it.' That was less of a problem than getting our senior managers not to tell the younger managers, 'Look, young man, don't question me.'

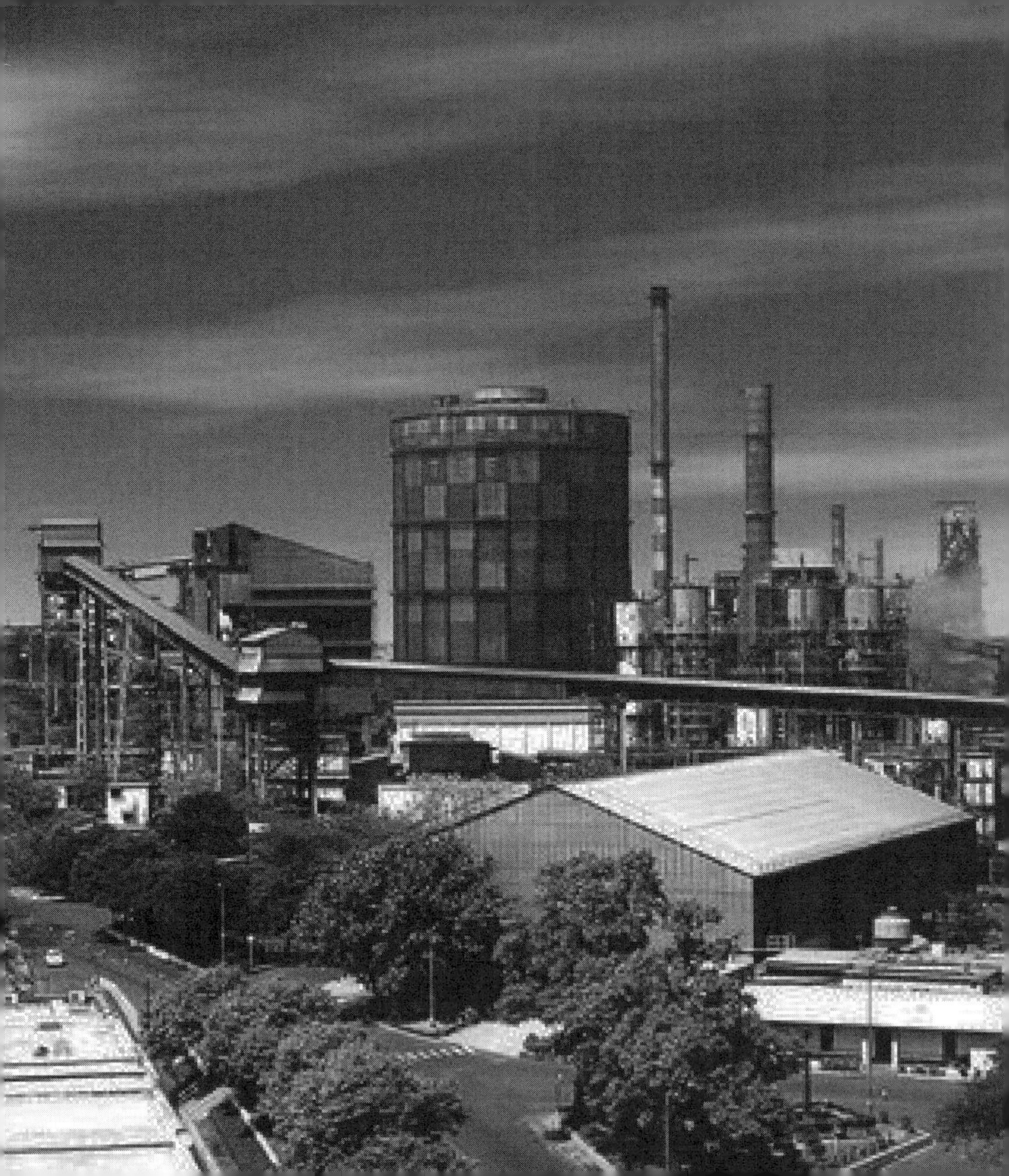

Without being critical, it is true that many of our companies had their heads in the sand and were resting on past glories. In the course of time, the view gained ground that we were less nimble than others, more resistant to change and more set in our ways. What we needed to do, of course, was benchmark ourselves against the best, get away from doing things the way we were, and put certain processes in place.

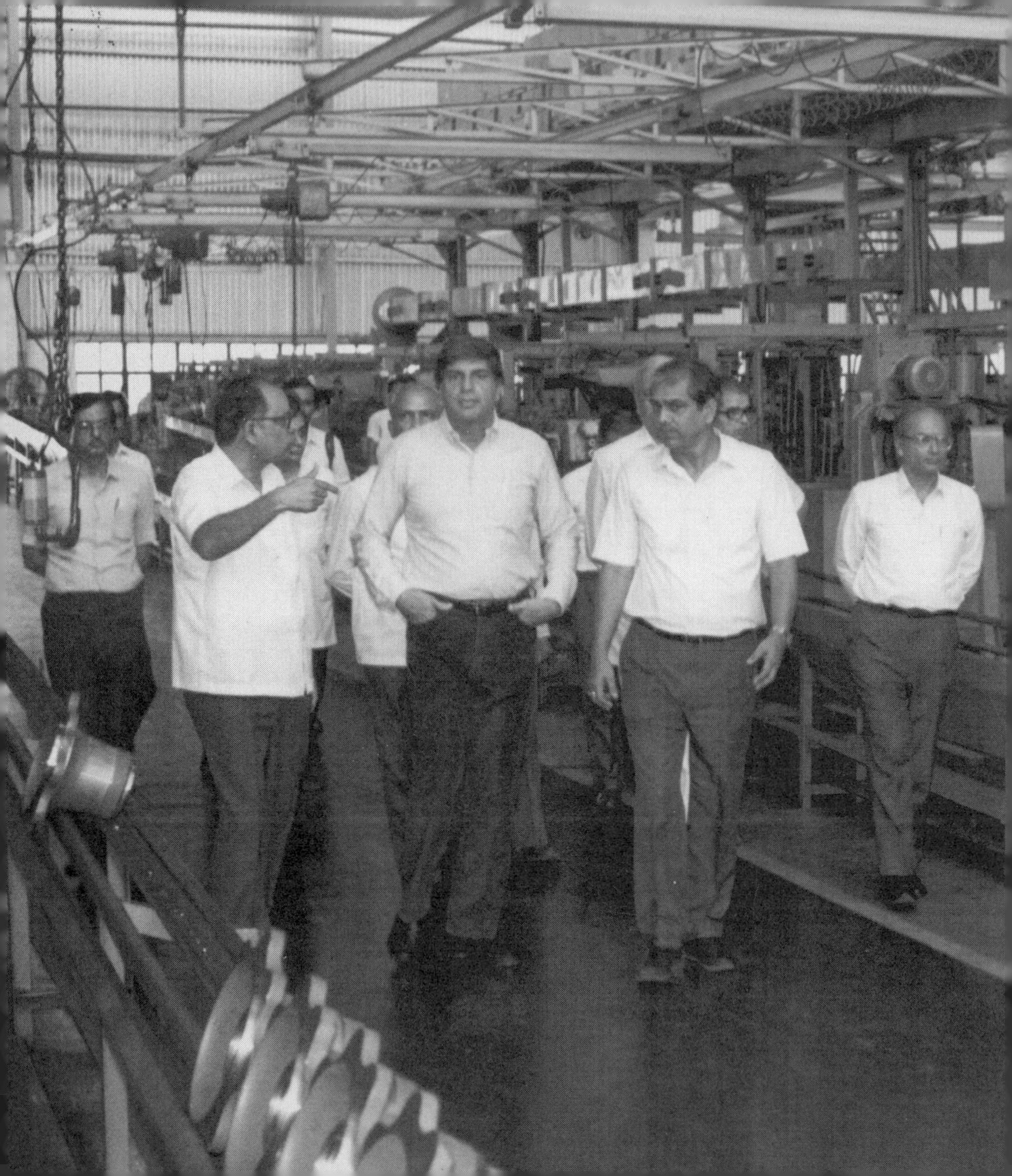

There was a need to refocus and look at how your customer sees you, and to pay more attention to what the customer wants, rather than what you think she wants. Are you really the most cost-effective producer? Are you aggressive enough to grab market share? Will you endeavour to dip your toe in the water and do something that you haven't done before?

We haven't been successful or innovative enough.

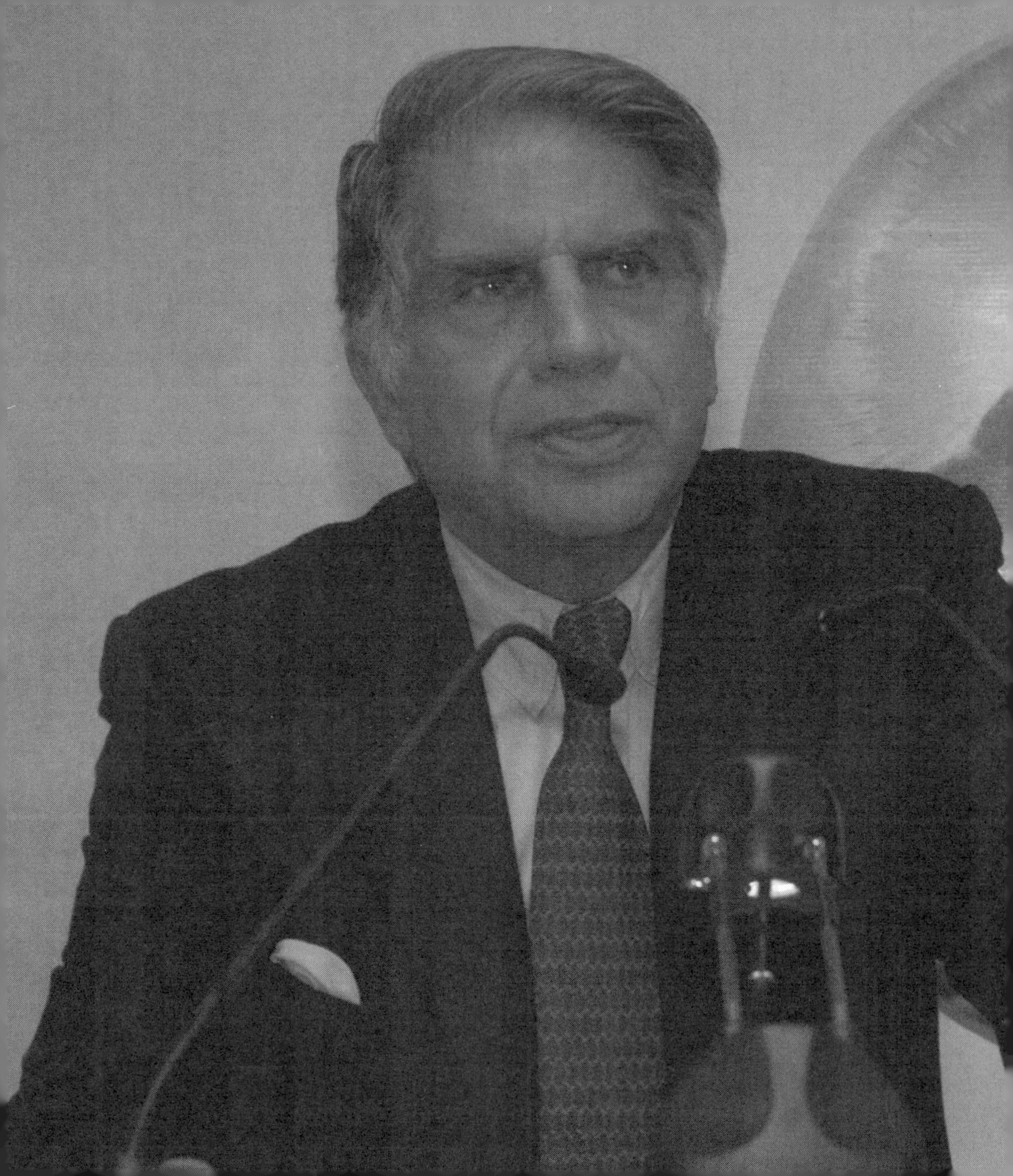

Sacrifices, loyalty and individual acts of heroism will always remain in my memory to reinforce the great sense of pride I have in having been a member of this team.

(From his farewell letter to Tata colleagues.)

THE TATA WAY

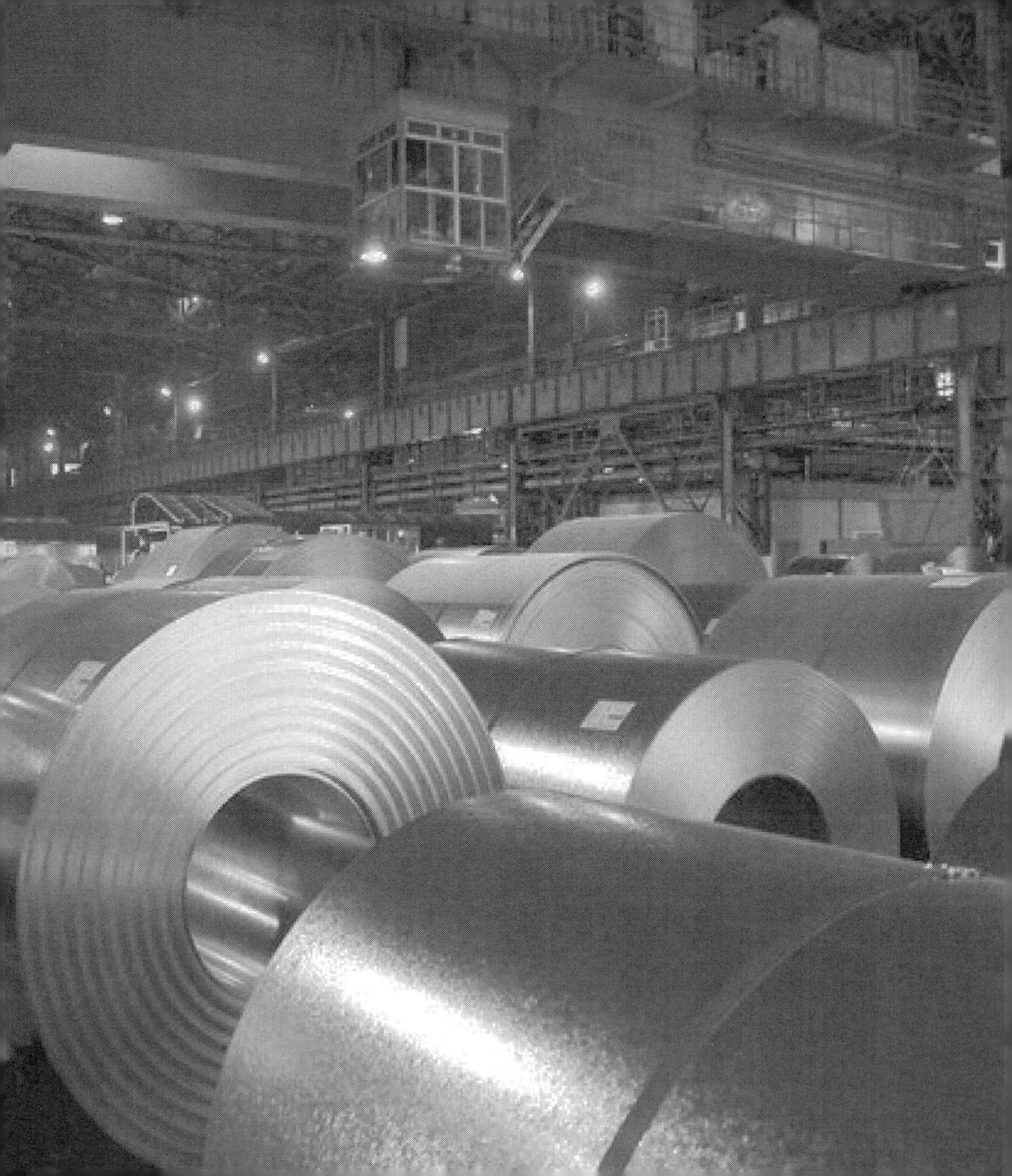

All companies need to keep looking at their business definition and, possibly from time to time, see if that needs to be redefined. For example, at Tata Steel they could say they are a steel company and find themselves in a shrinking market where steel is under threat of being replaced by some other material. The question is: what do we call ourselves? One view was that steel is a material, so can we be a materials company? We don't have to be in all materials, but can we be in composites, can we be in plastics, laminates, etc? The automotive business needs to think similarly. We have to keep looking at ourselves and asking: what is our business?

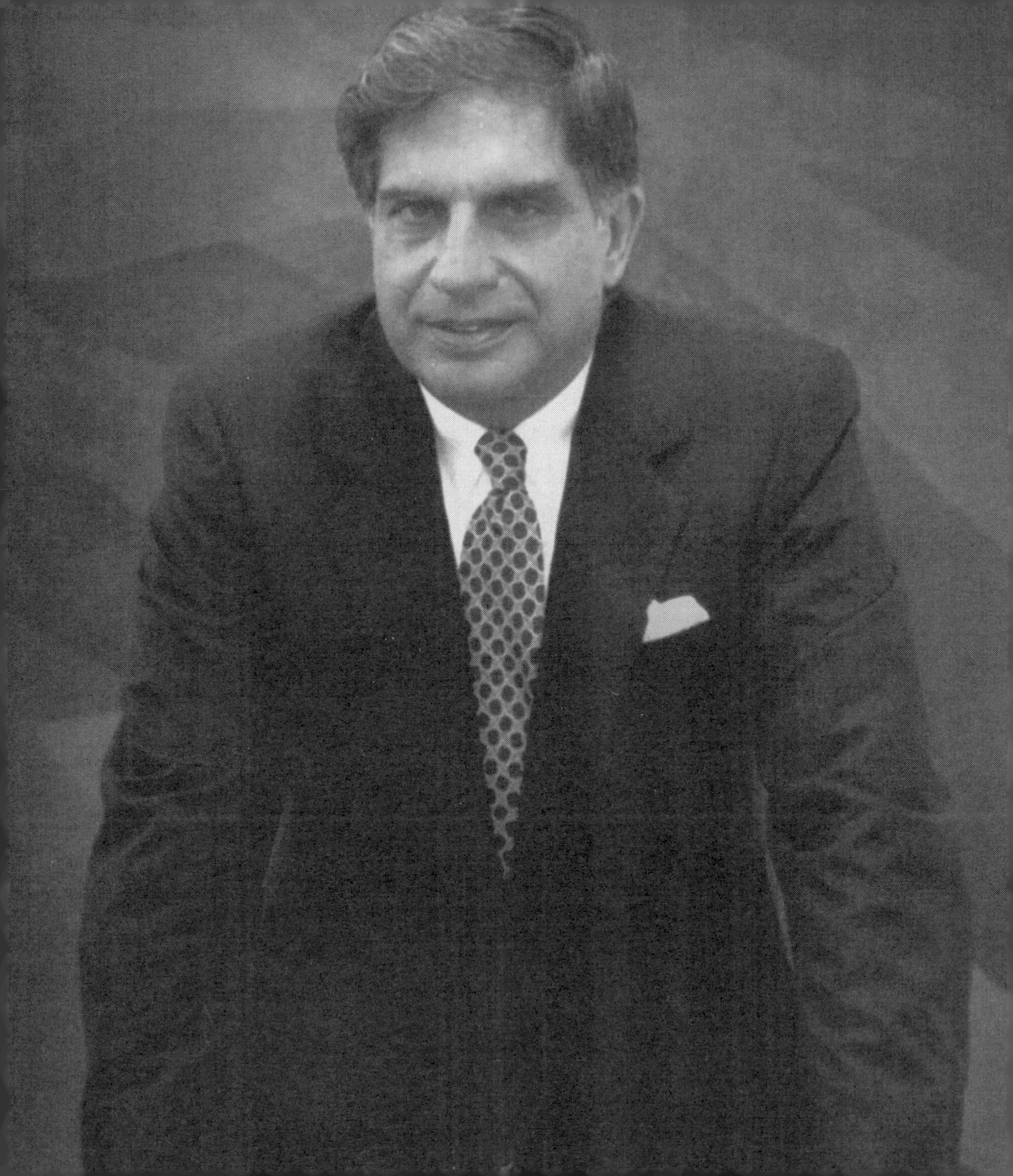

Today the world does not afford you the luxury of being a slow mover. We have to be aggressive and farsighted enough to look into the future, and we also have to be pragmatic enough to say that if we really are not in a leadership position in a particular business, we should look at exiting that business.

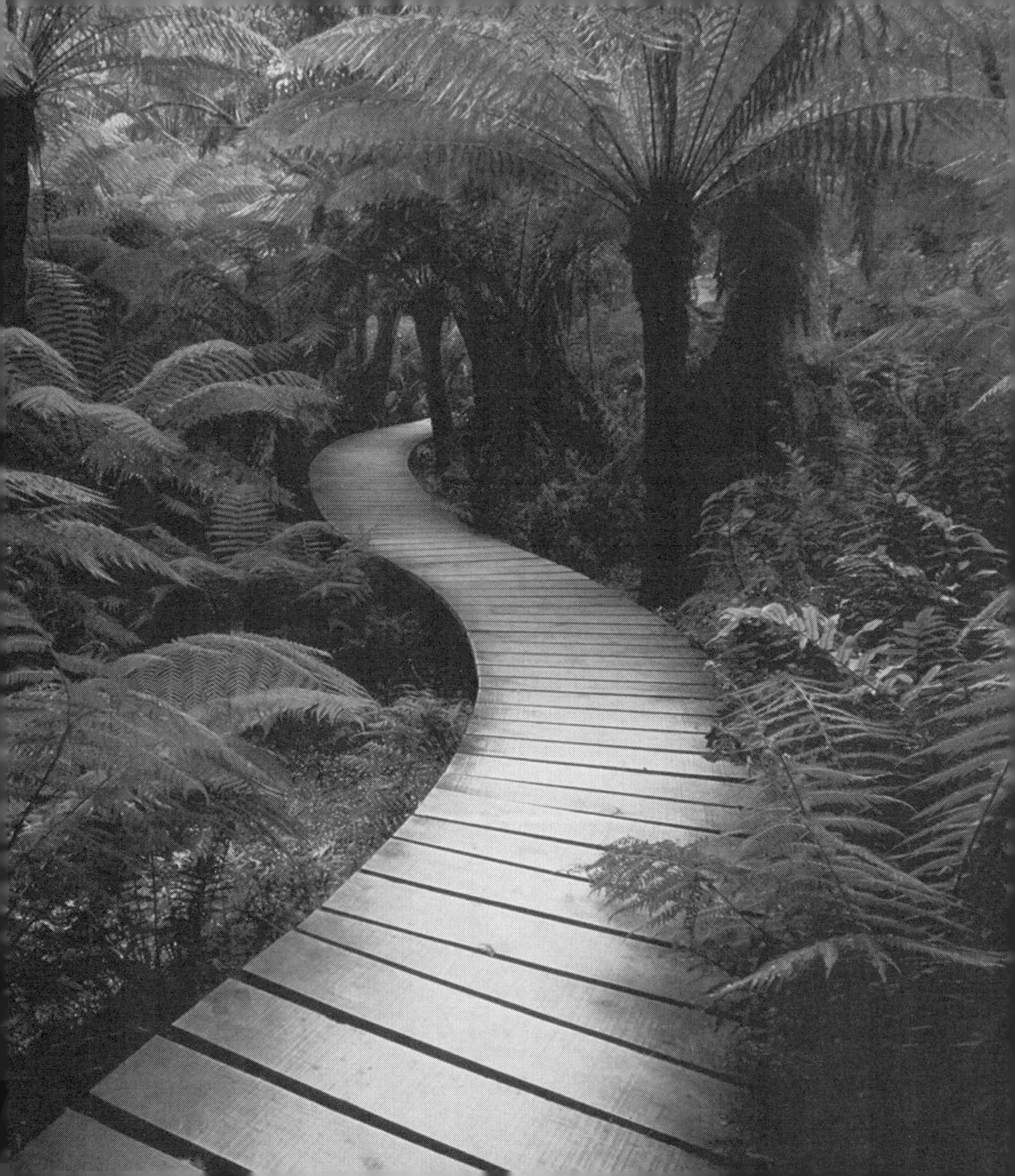

We at the Tata group have to be creative on the basis of our strengths: low costs, technological richness, innovation.

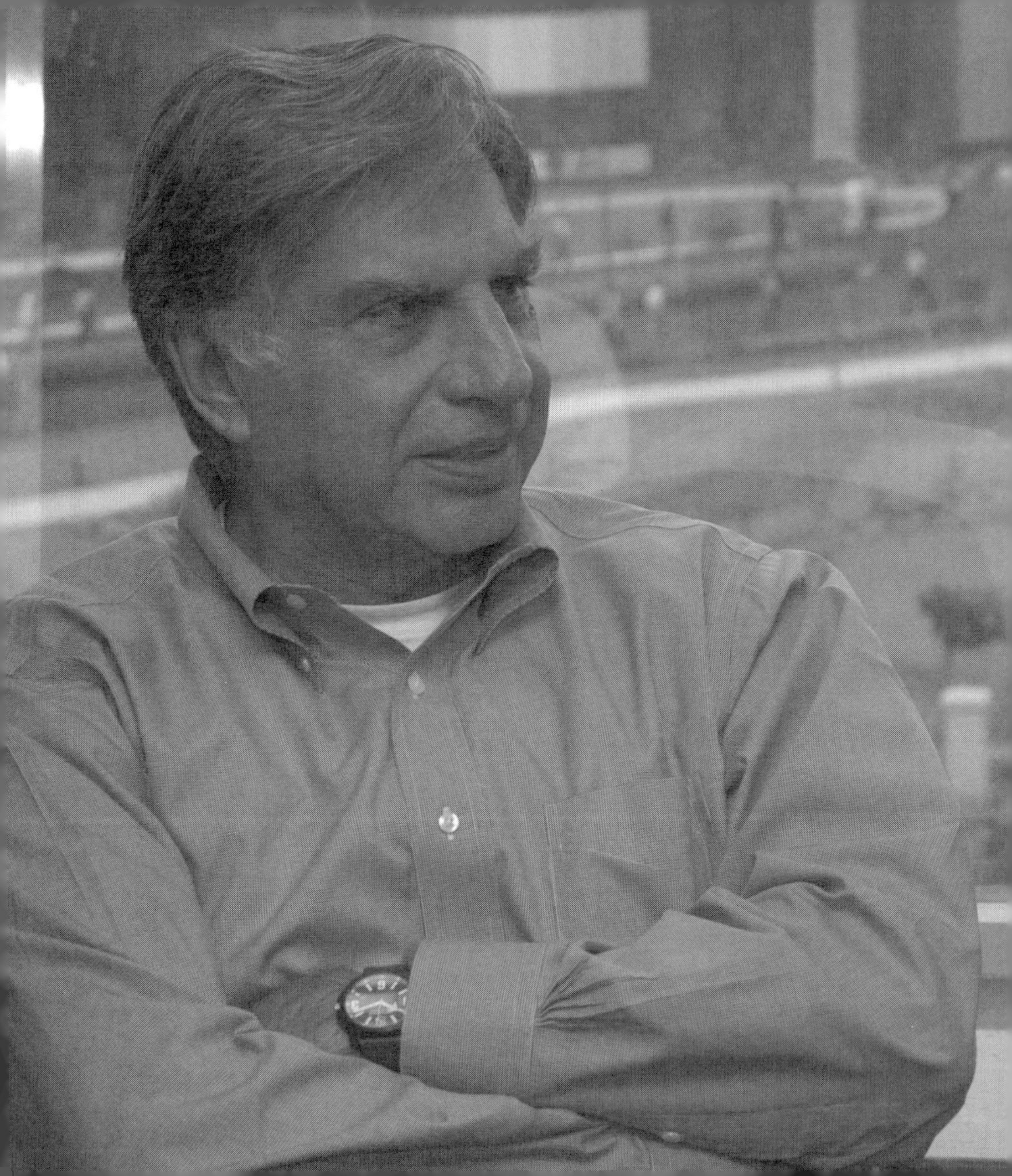

The kind of company one would want to emulate is one where products and technology are at the leading edge, dealings with customers are very fair, services are of a high order, and business ethics are transparent and straightforward. A less tangible issue involves the work environment, which should not be one where you are stressed and driven to the point of being drugged.

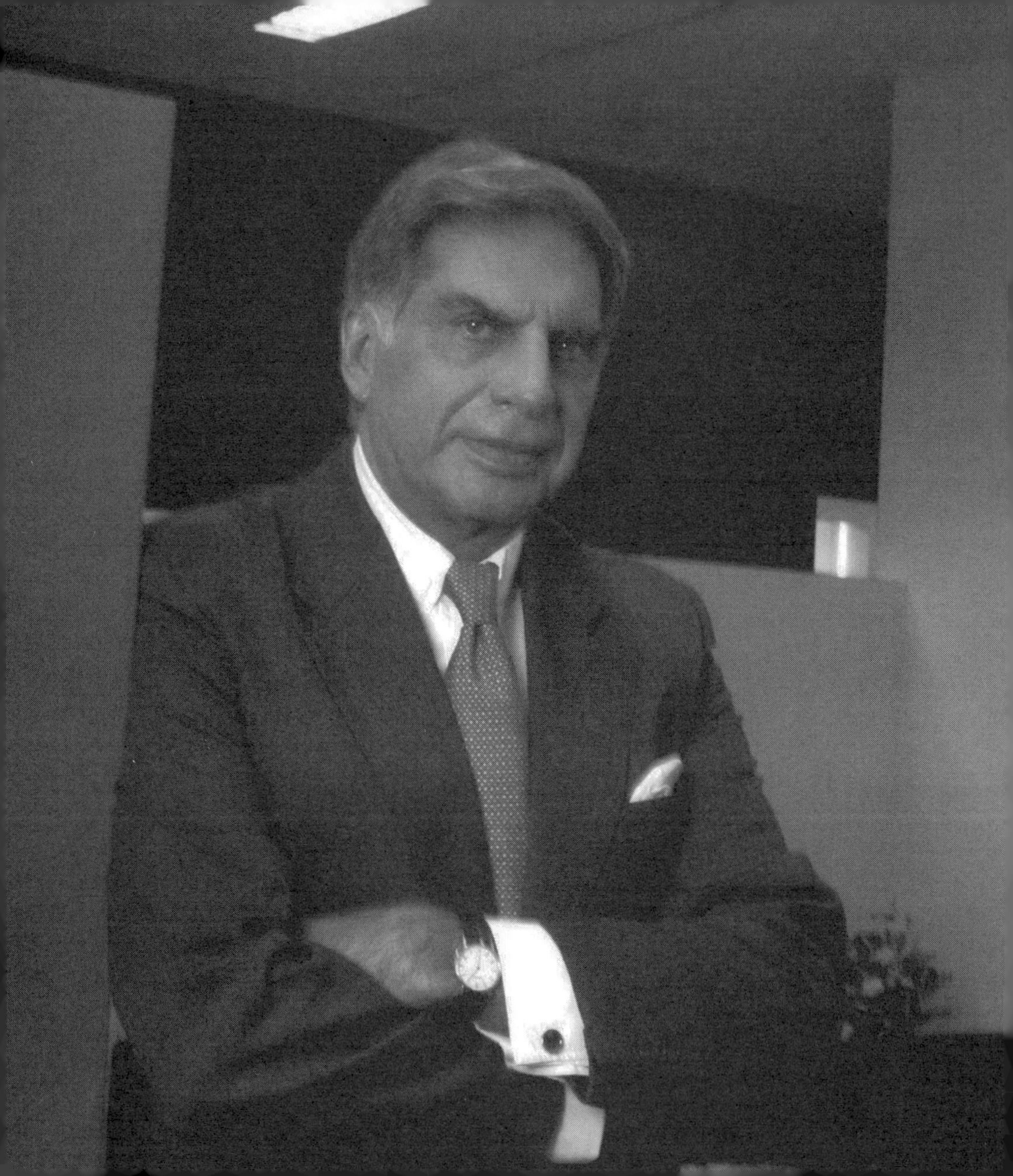

The way to retain employees today is to make their work and their day-to-day activities in the company exciting enough for them to stay. Not everyone will stay, but I think we can empower more people if we are willing to pass on the responsibility for that. If people are satisfied and motivated, there's less chance of them wanting to leave and go to a competitor.

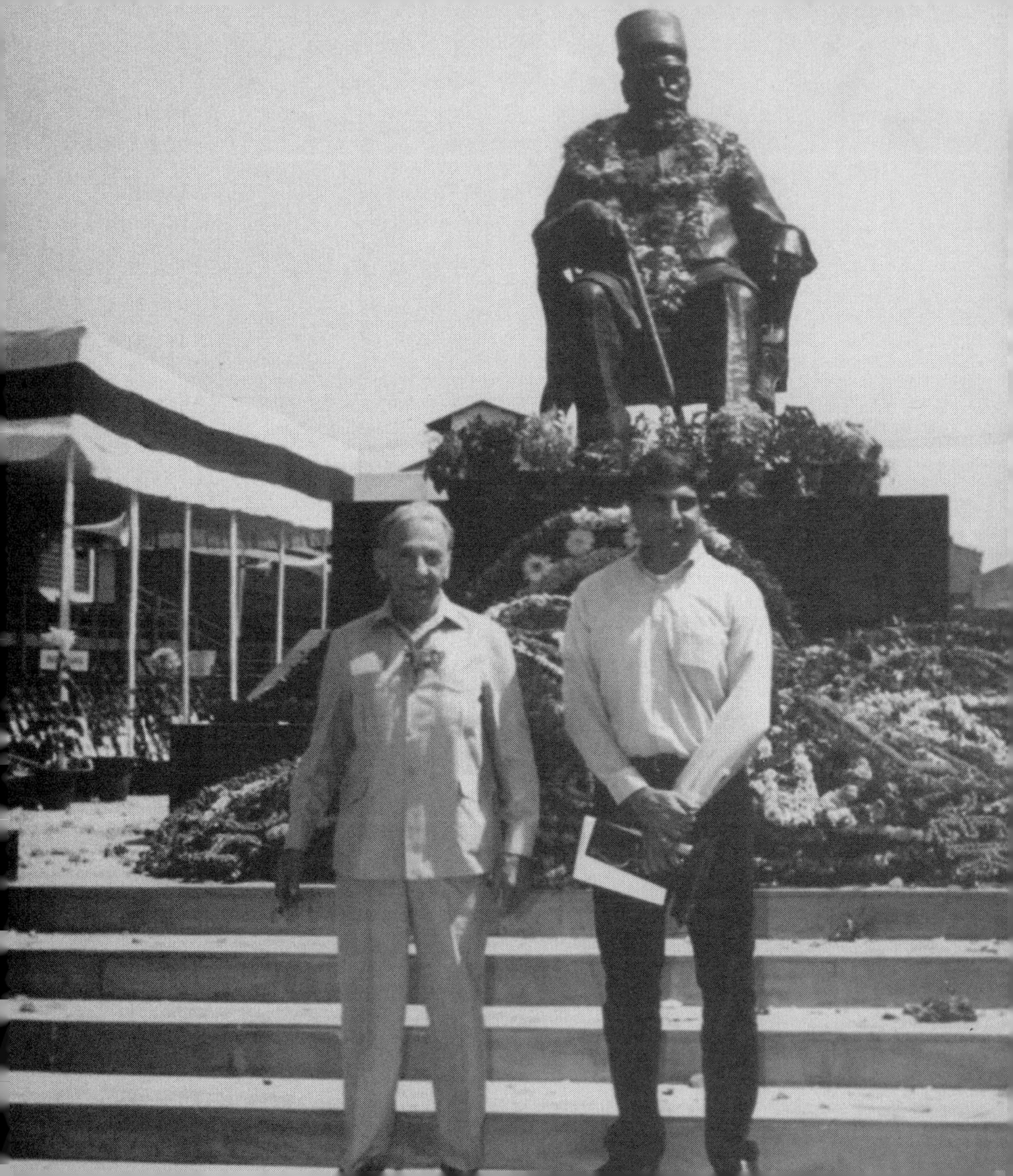

The Tatas have to be less risk-averse. We have been a very conservative house and we have been applauded for our conservatism, but today we need to take more risk. We don't need to be flamboyant or cavalier, but we need to be less conservative than we have been.

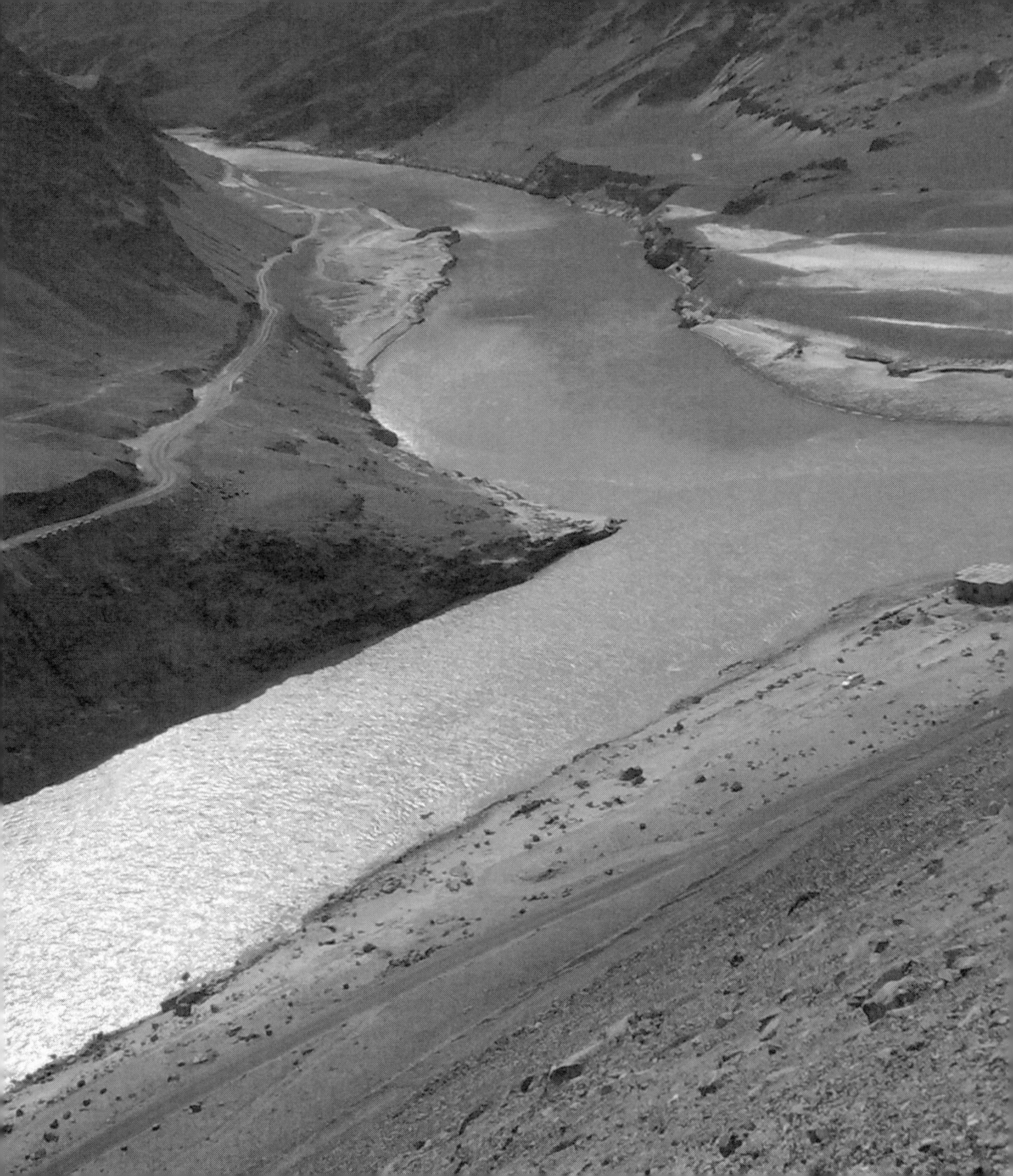

The Tata group must lead India in terms of what it does, not only in business but also as a corporate citizen and as a participant in the country's growth. This is a holistic view. We want our managers and companies to drive their businesses using every means they can to achieve their ends, but they must do it in a way which stands out and continues the traditions that the group has established over the years.

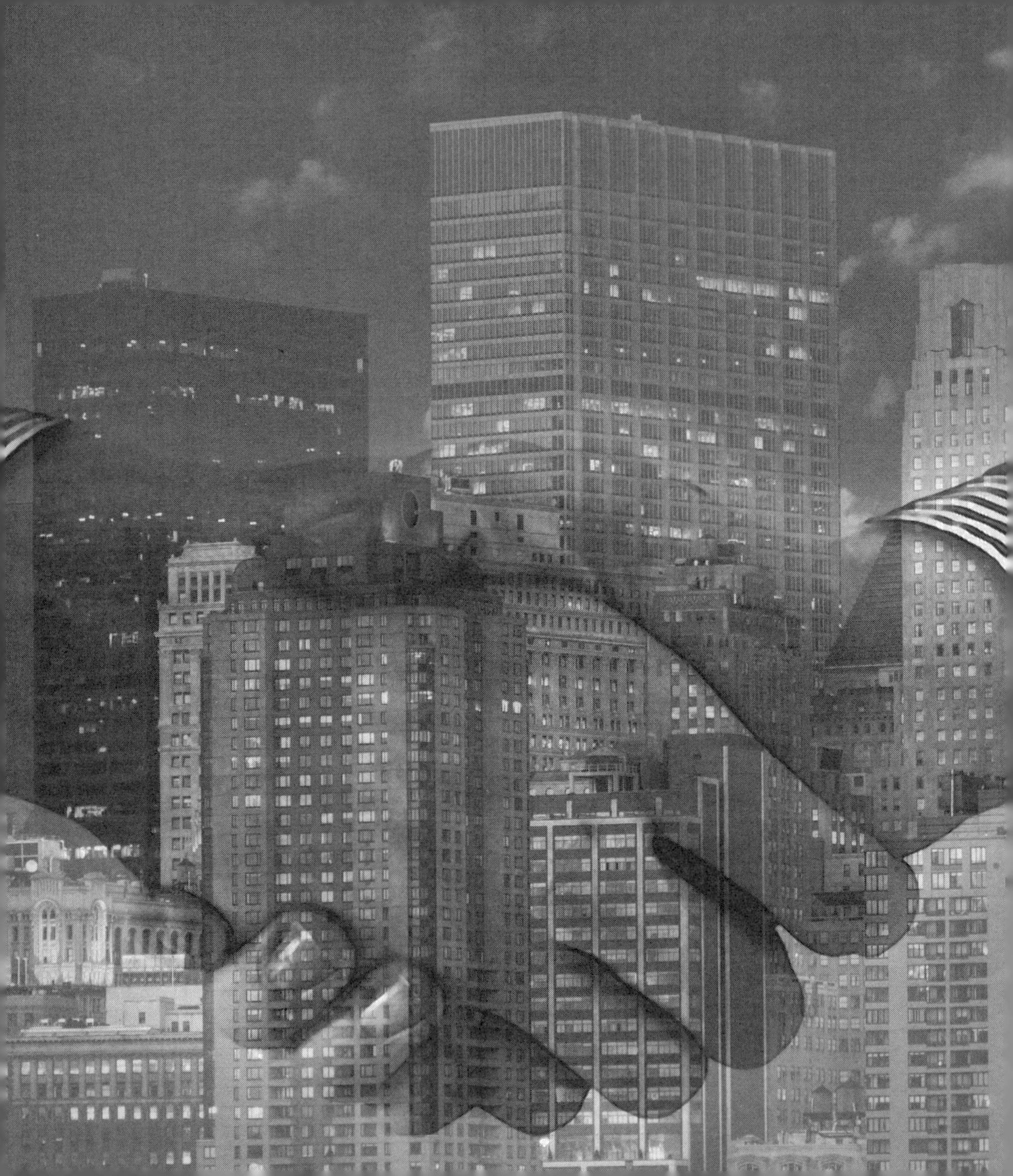

We should be treating the customer in the same way that we would want to be treated as customers.

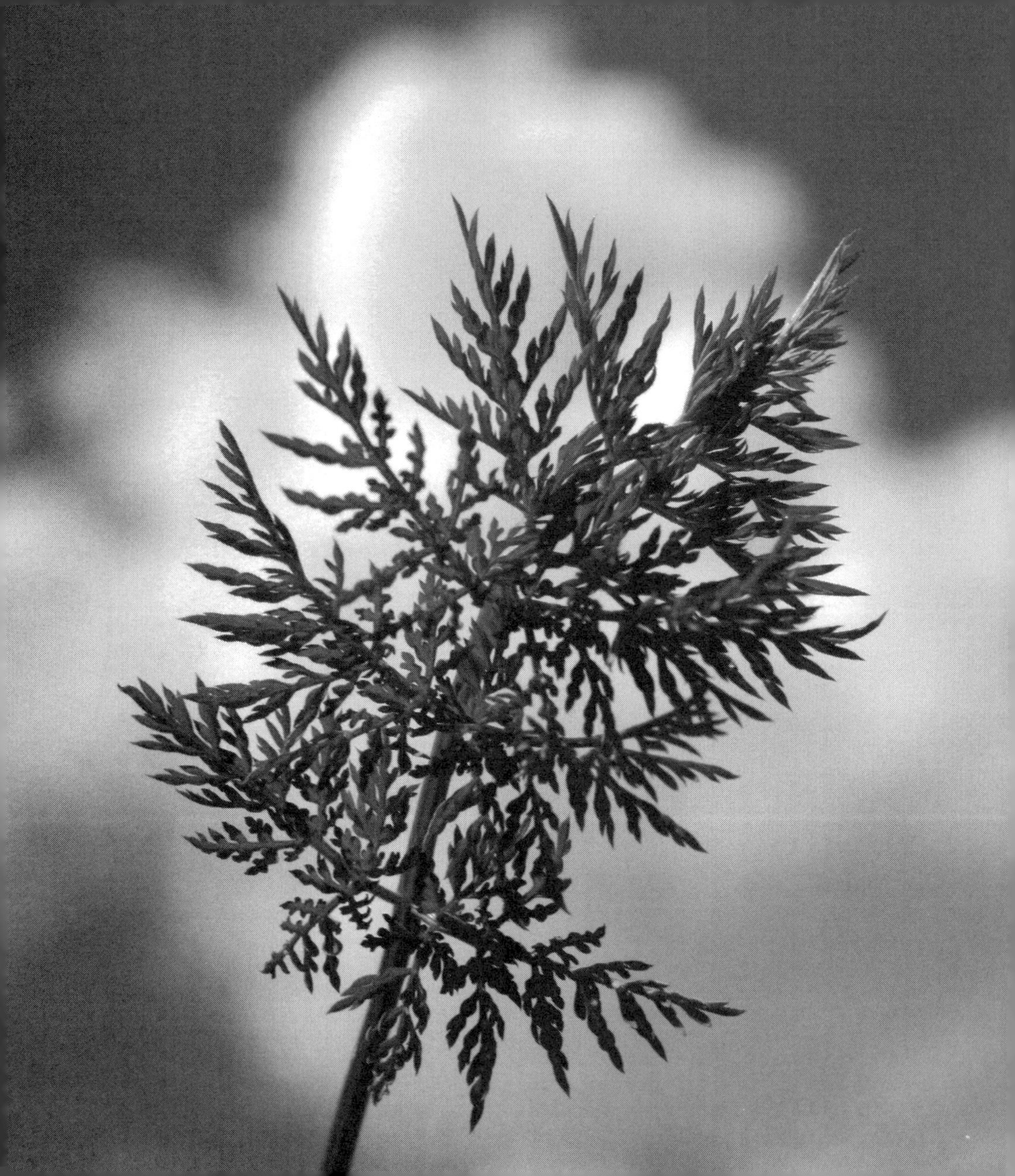

Where we have direct dealings with our customers, it is important that they are shown courtesy, dealt with fairly, and made to feel that they are receiving the attention they deserve. The interface with the customer should be a seamless one.

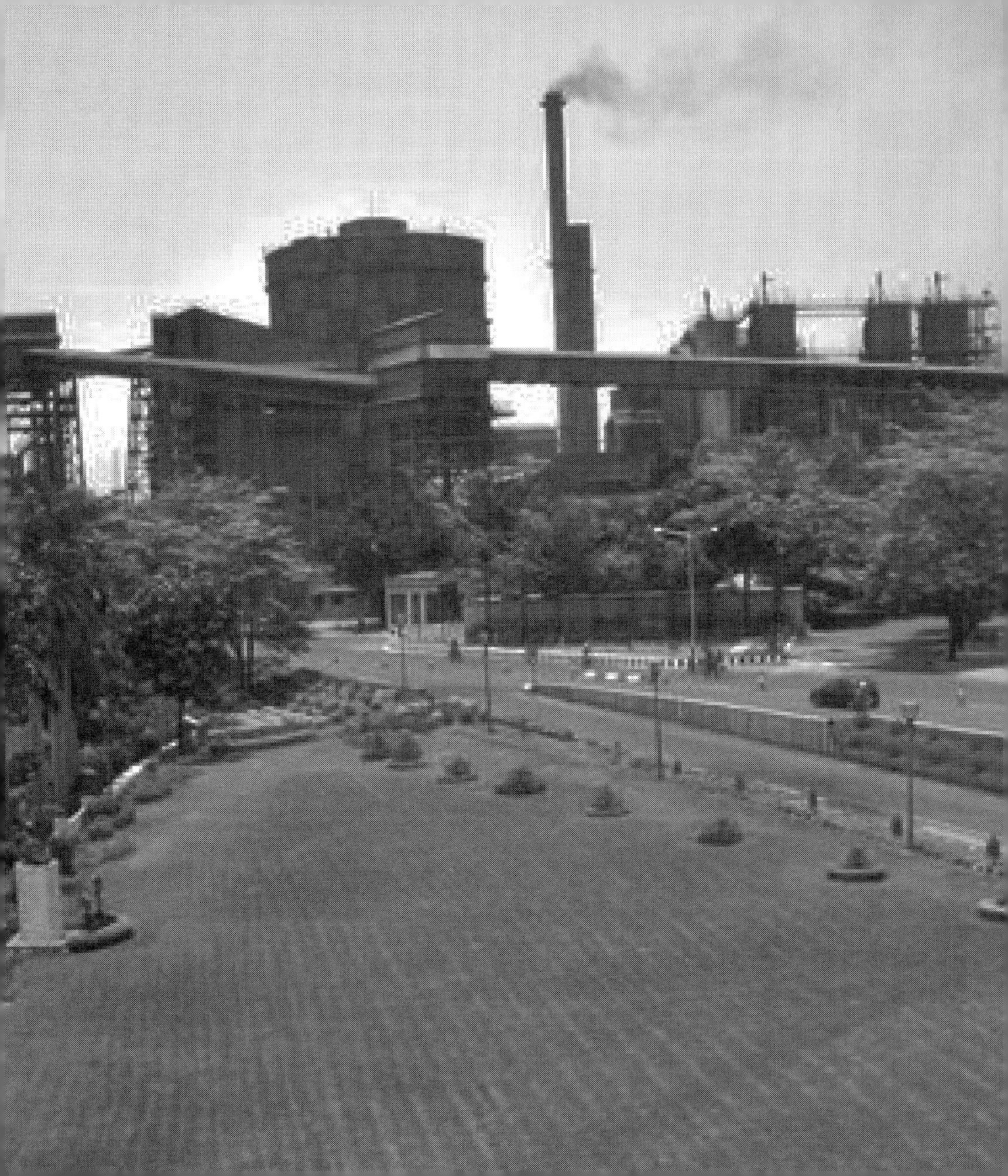

It should not be, cannot be, that low-cost products come to mean inferior or substandard products and services; definitely not. The aim is to create products for that larger segment, good and robust products that we are able to produce innovatively and get to the marketplace at a lower cost.

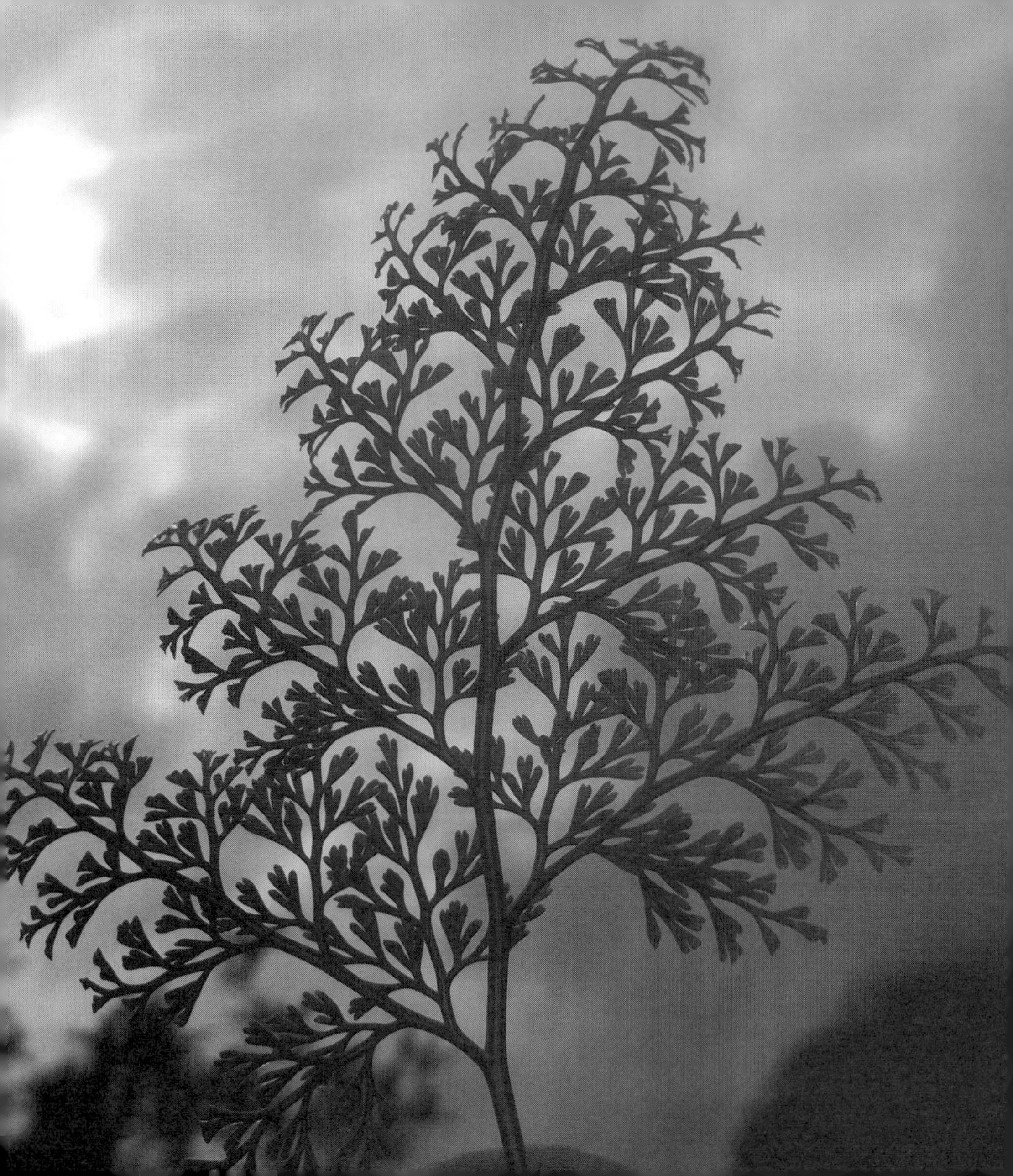

We did everything in small increments, so we always lagged behind. But the crucial question is: can we venture putting a man on the moon or risk billions of rupees on a really way-out, advanced project in, say, superconductors? Do you restrict your risk to something close to your heart?

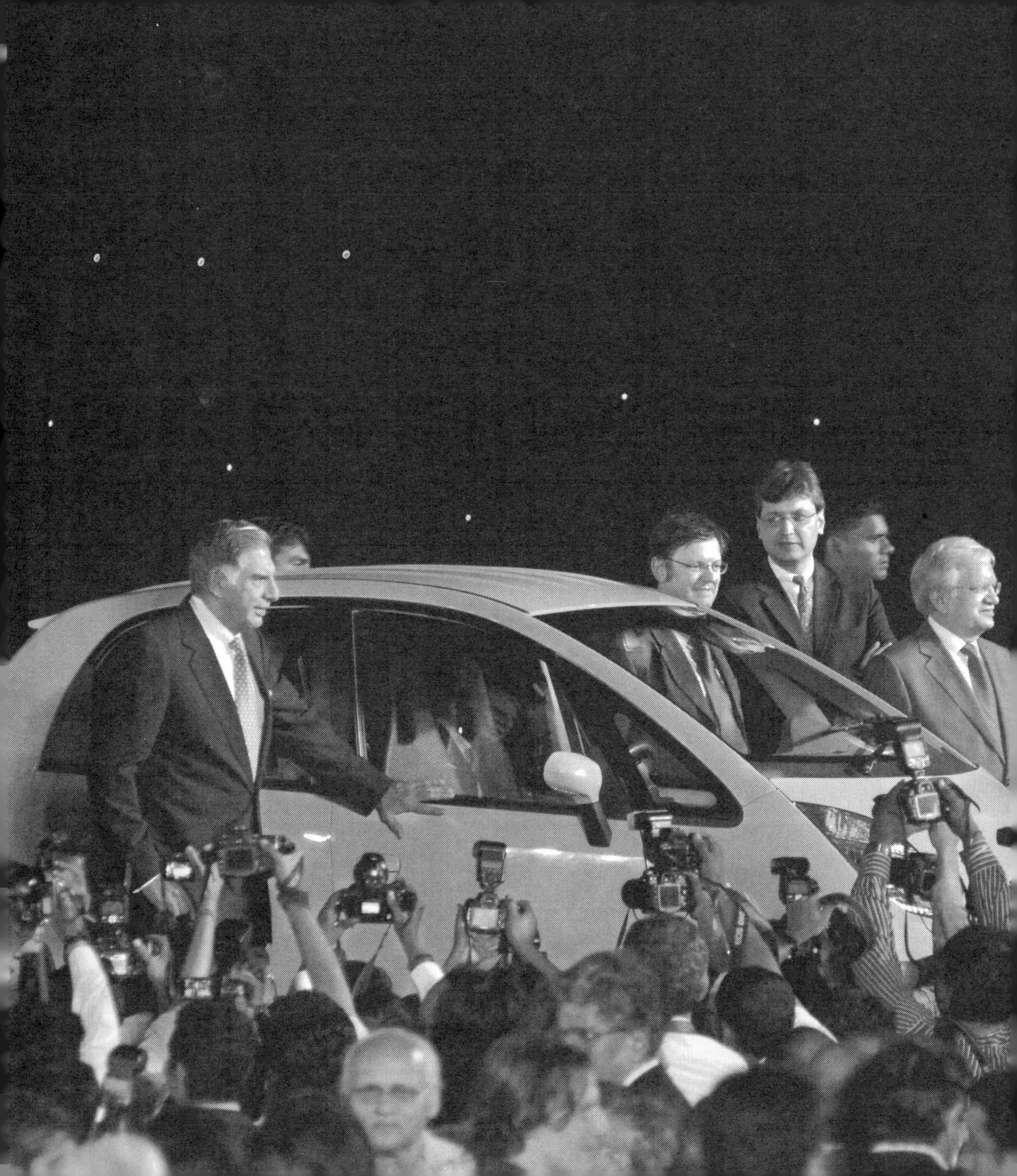

My outlook on R&D is that it is an absolutely necessary thing for us to do. And I don't think we are doing enough. The point is not just spending money; it's how many patents you file, your innovation rate and your product development… If today you were to give everybody a mandate that they can spend 3 per cent of their revenue on R&D, assuming they can spare the money, I don't think many companies would know the what, where and how of spending that kind of money, other than to put up some infrastructure and buy lots of equipment.

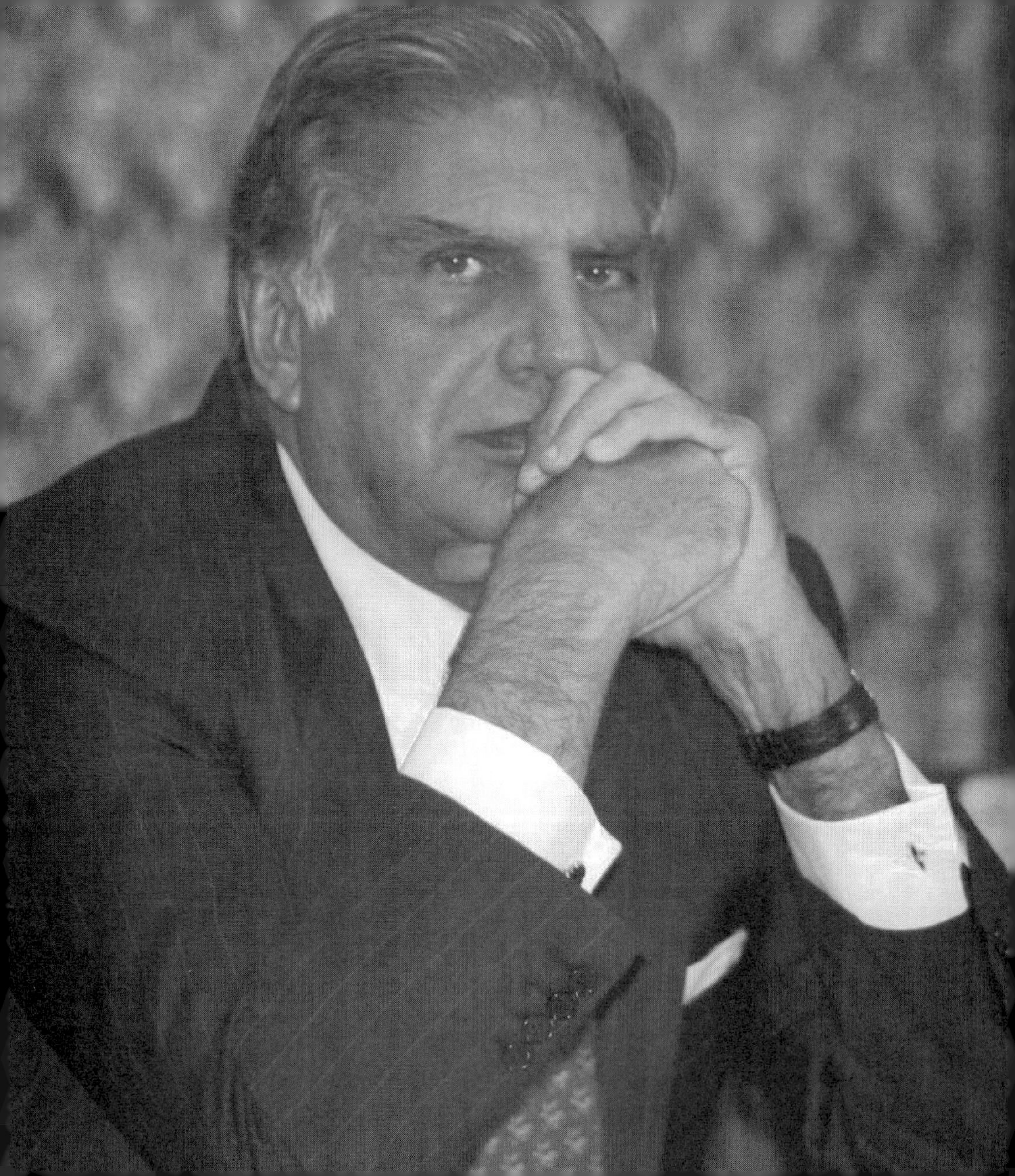

We have to clamp down on deviations from commitments. To ensure greater commitment to performance, we also need to have a system which rewards performers and punishes those who don't perform.

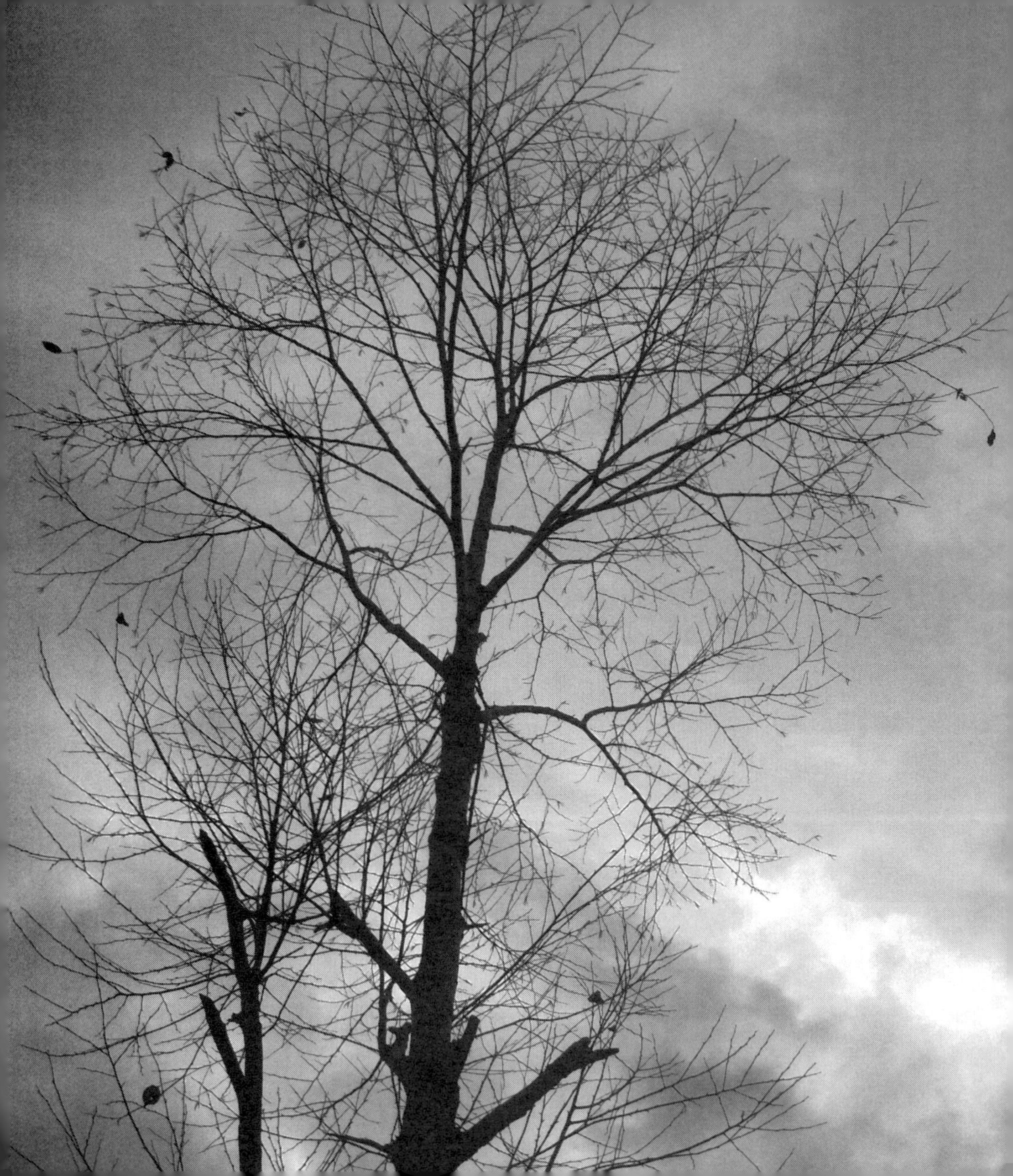

What we do when somebody breaks the code, how we deal with that person, I think that is the true index of our behaviour. When we have had a rogue officer or director, we have actually prosecuted that person and the person has gone to jail.

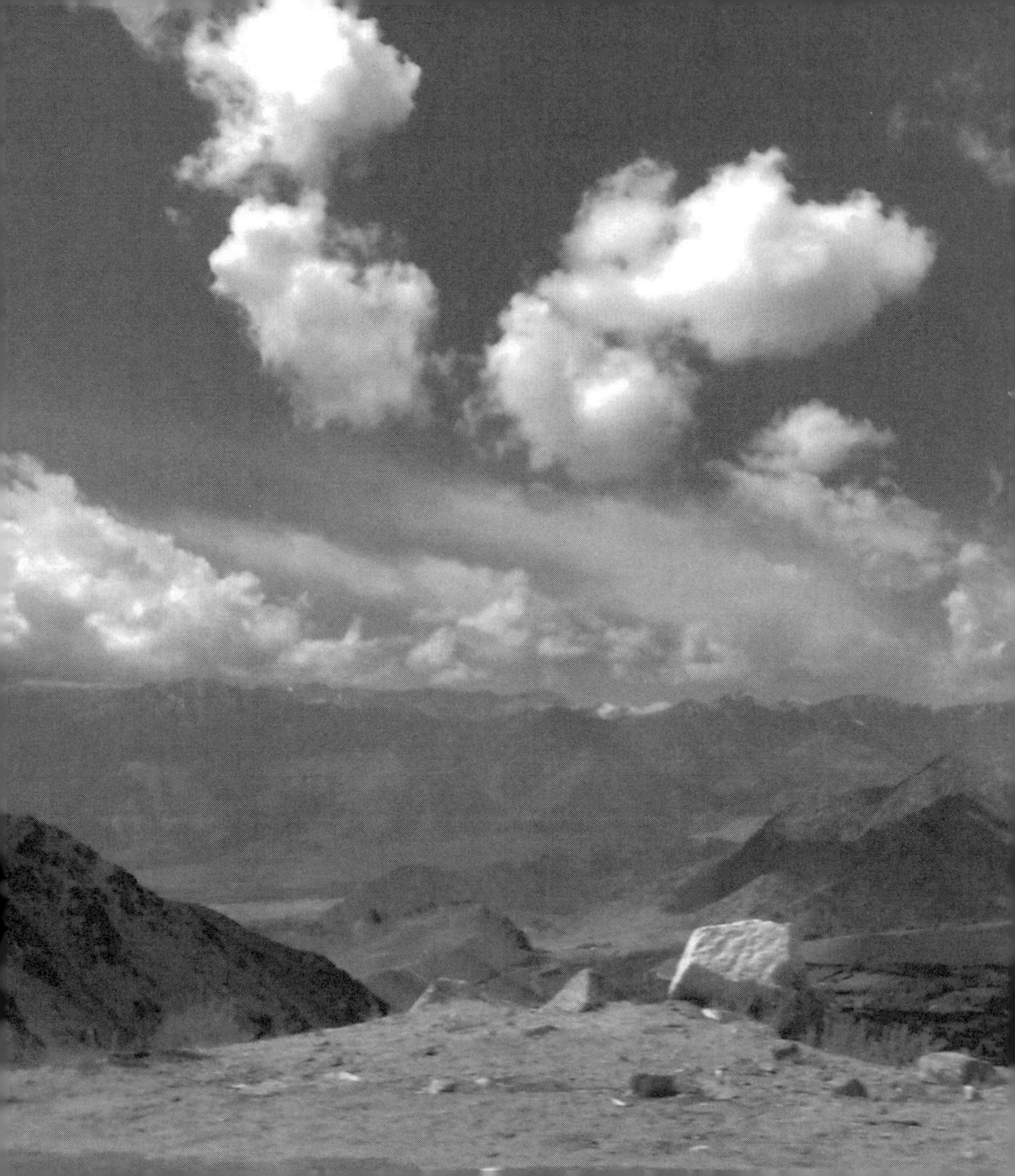

One big challenge is being globally competitive. This may be a function of scale or product design, but the critical question is: can we be globally competitive in giving the customer a product equal to or better than what he or she already has access to? The other is: can we be technologically advanced enough?

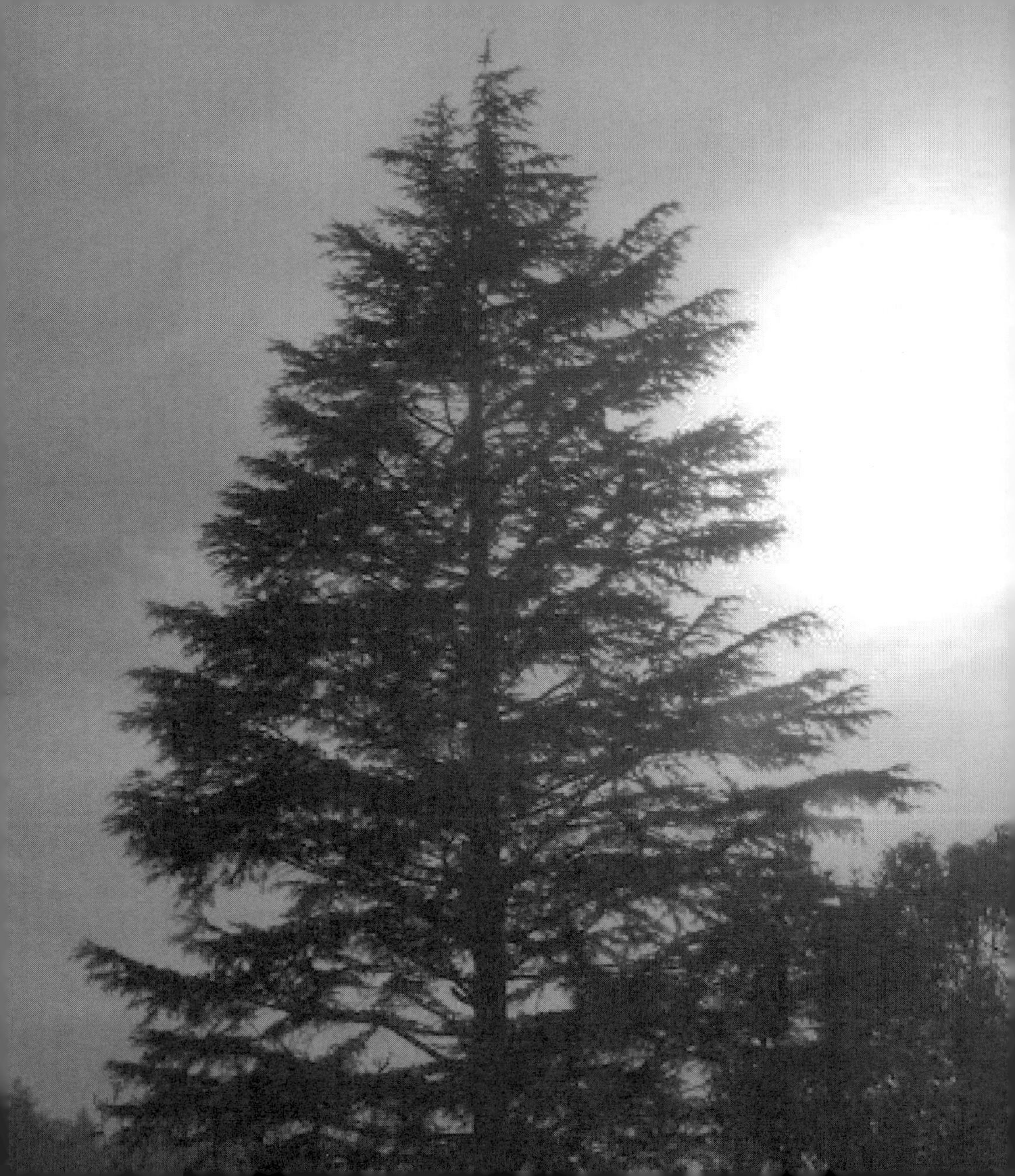

What we do before we acquire a company is spend a lot of time looking at the human chemistry, its management and work ethics, and the manner of working of that company.

TATA

Leadership with Trust

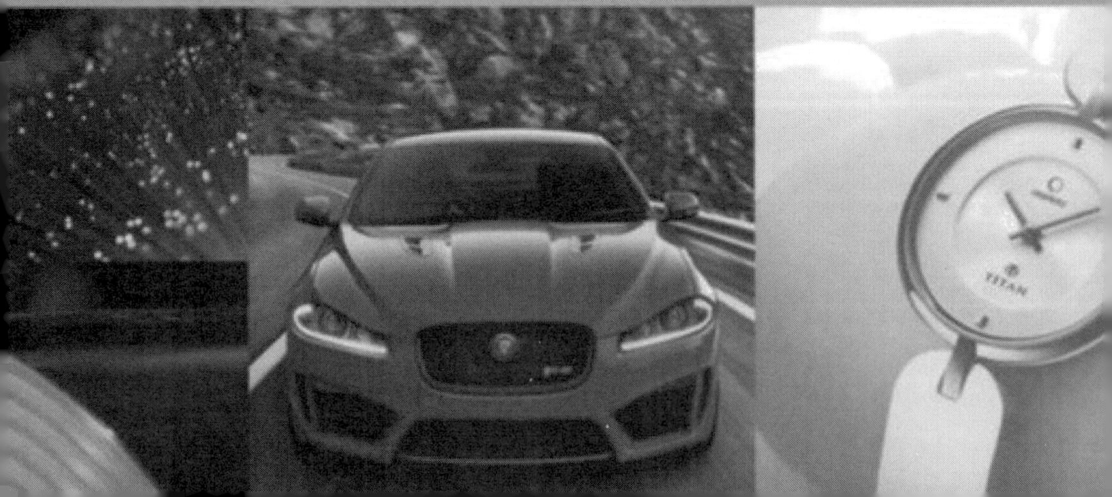

We are probably not doing enough to build the Tata brand globally, but we are one of the most recognisable corporate names coming out of India. Apart from size, market capitalisation and the rest, we are seen as a poster boy for ethical business, trustworthy and fair. That's a model western companies feel comfortable with.

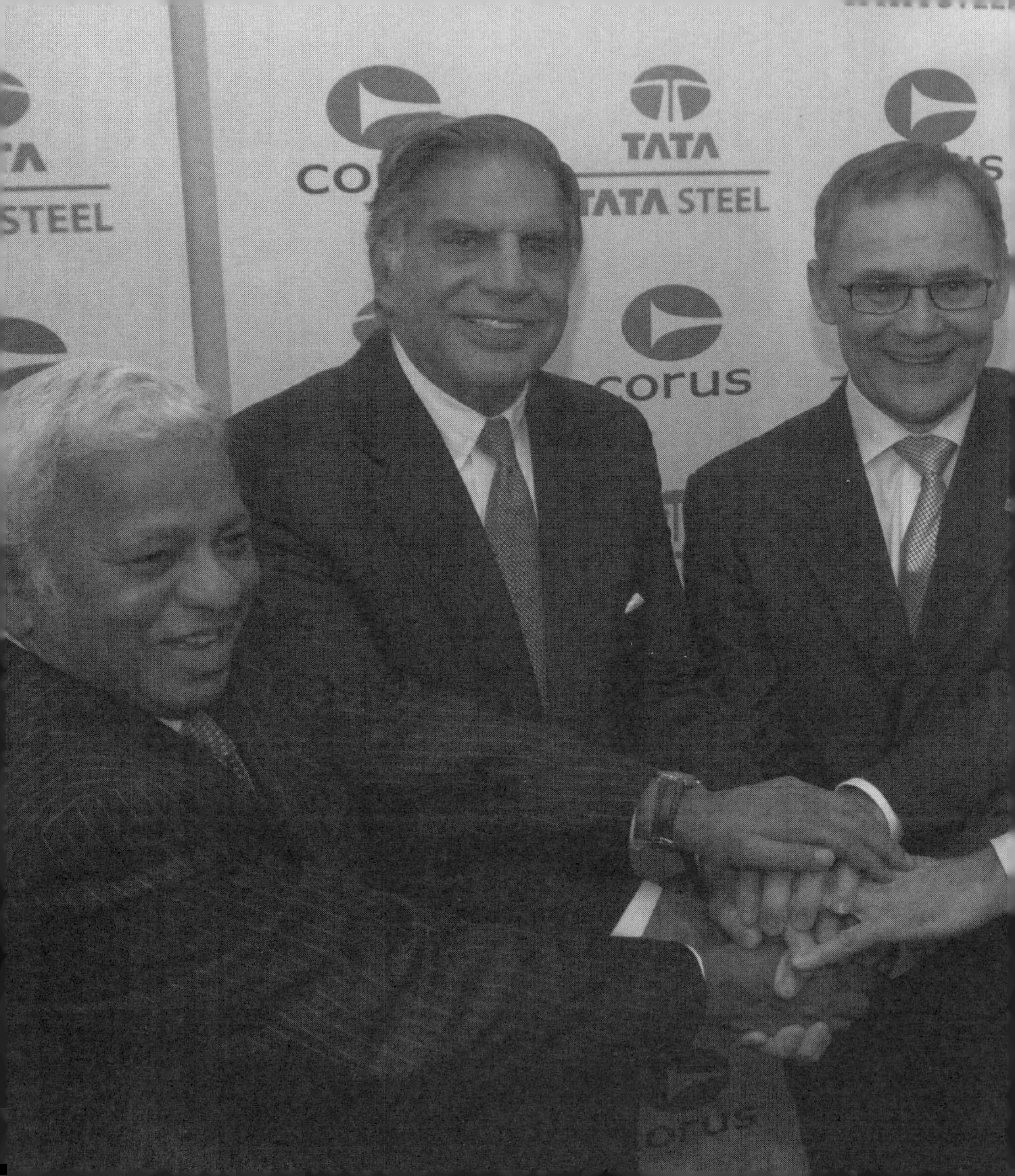
TATA
TATA STEEL
corus

It would be great if we were considered abroad as a globally operating company with a local touch, one that just happens to be owned by a group of Indians.

TATA

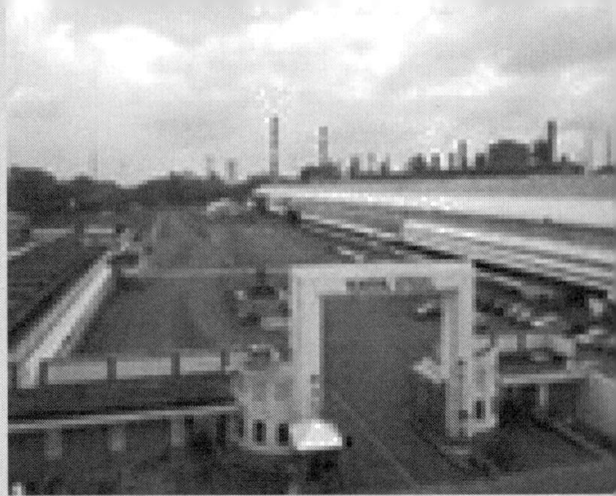

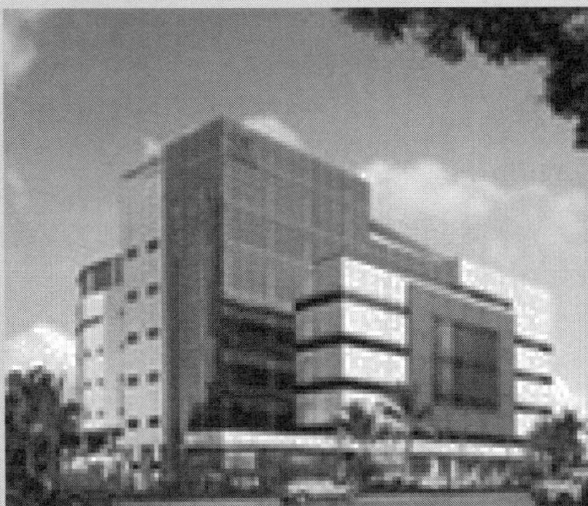

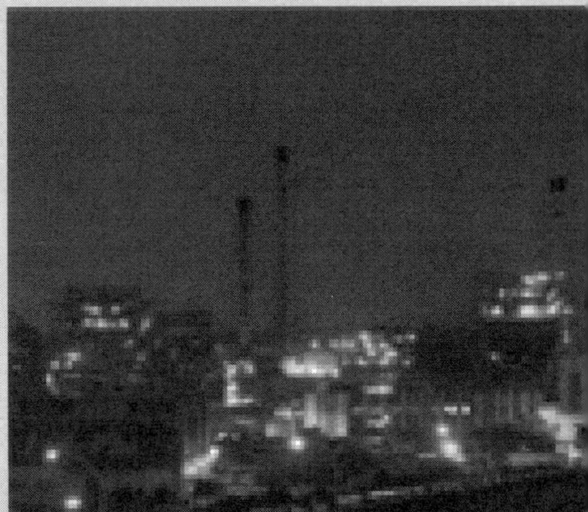

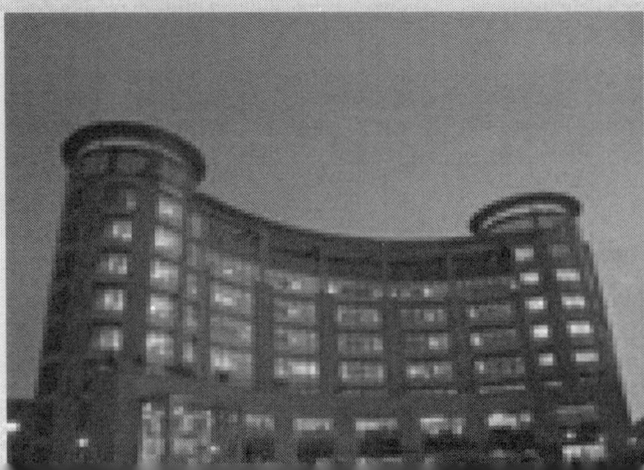

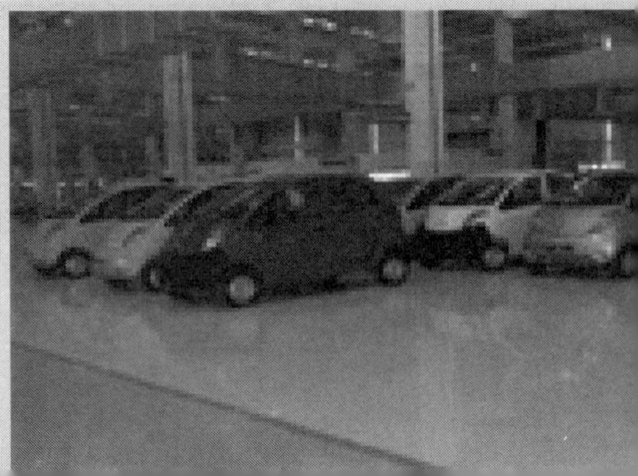

One hundred years from now, I expect the Tatas to be much bigger than they are now. More importantly, I hope the group comes to be regarded as being the best in India; best in the manner in which we operate, best in the products we deliver, and best in our value systems and ethics.

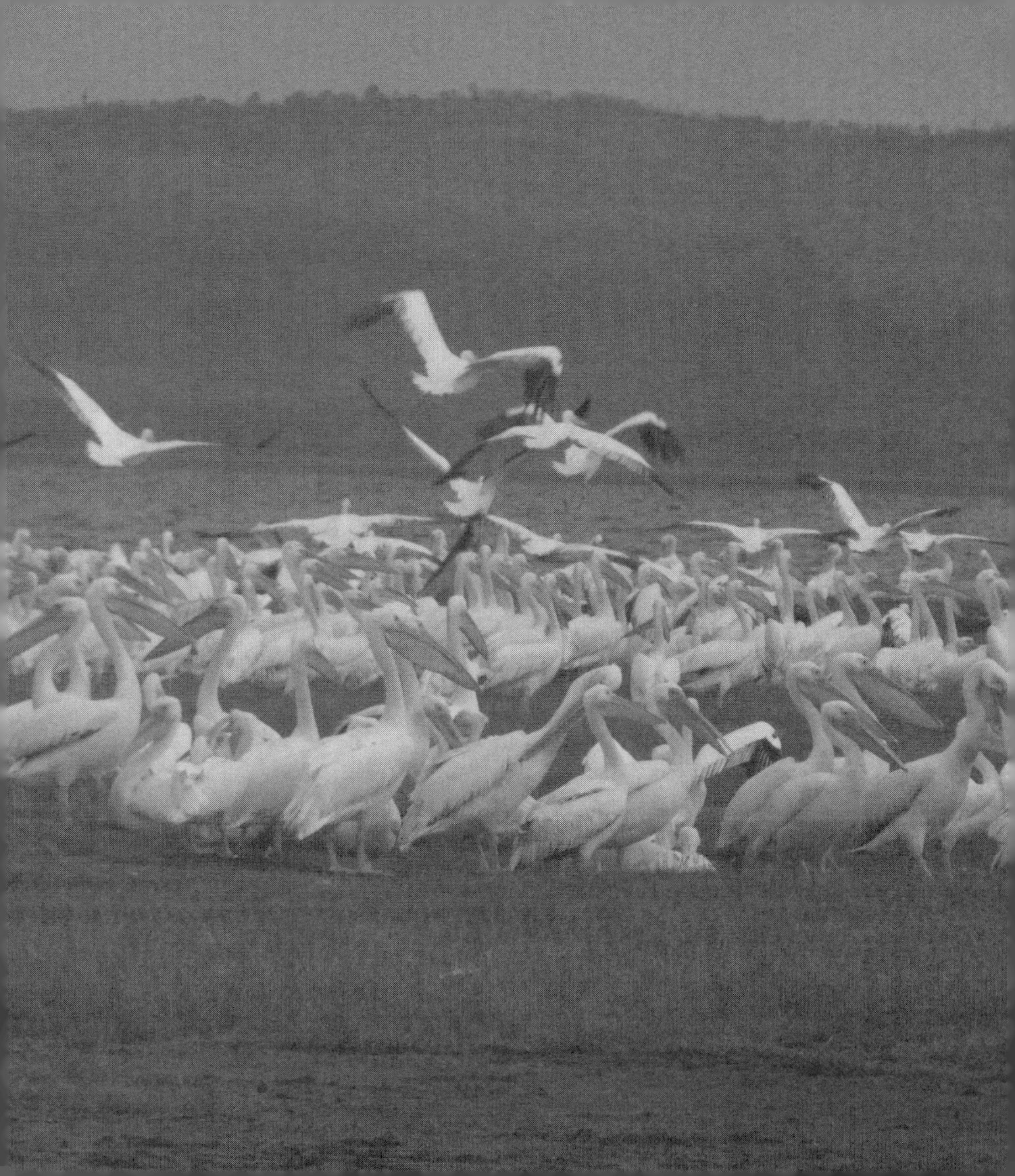

I expect that we will spread our wings far beyond India, that we will become a global group, operating in many countries, an Indian business conglomerate that is at home in the world, carrying the same sense of trust that we do today.

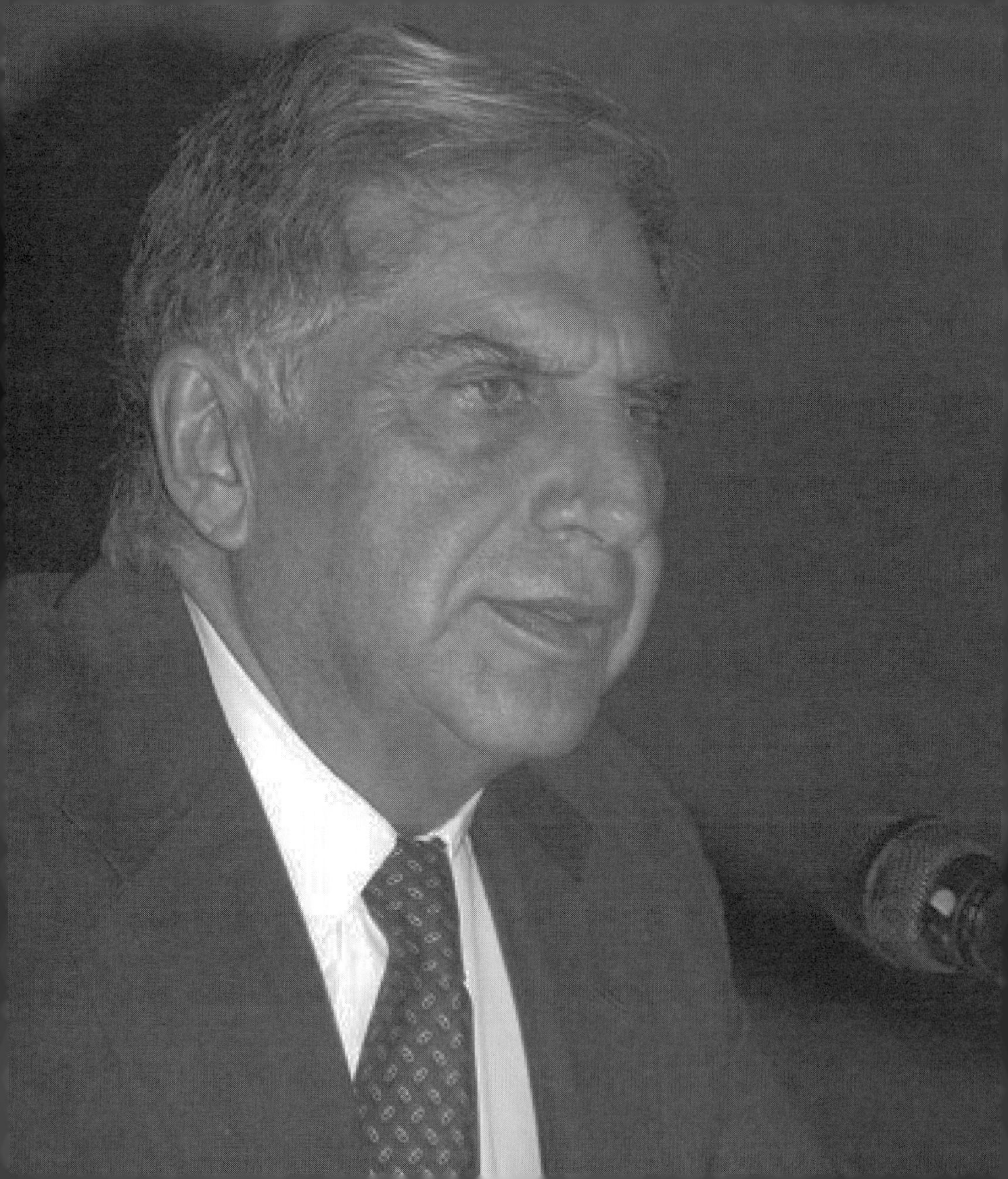

It is easy to become a number one player but it is difficult to remain number one. So we will have to fight with a view to remain number one.

THE NANO

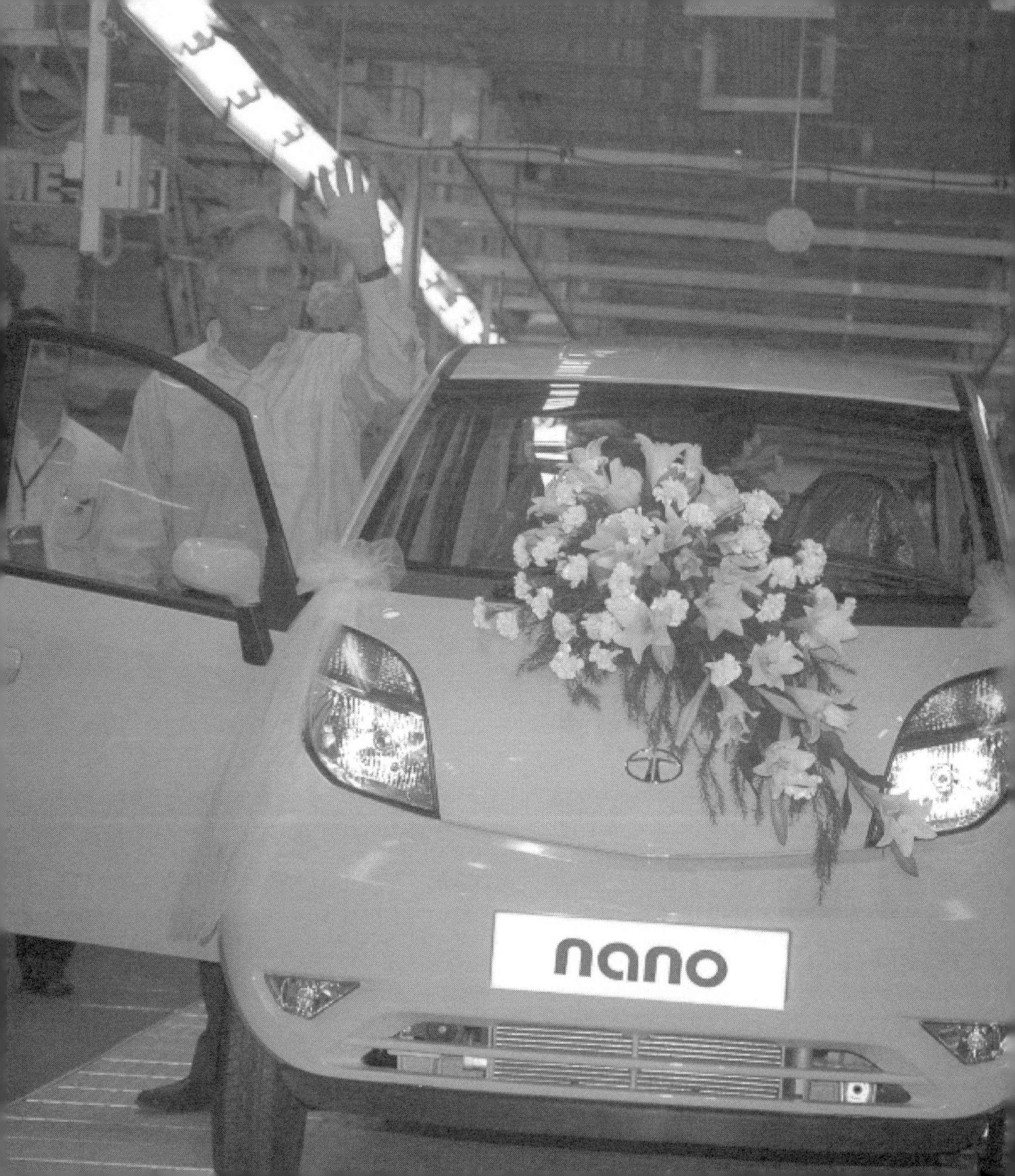
nano

A man on a two-wheeler with a child standing in front, his wife sitting behind. Add to that the wet roads and a family in potential danger. I hope to contribute to making life safer for them.

(Nano launch, December 2008)

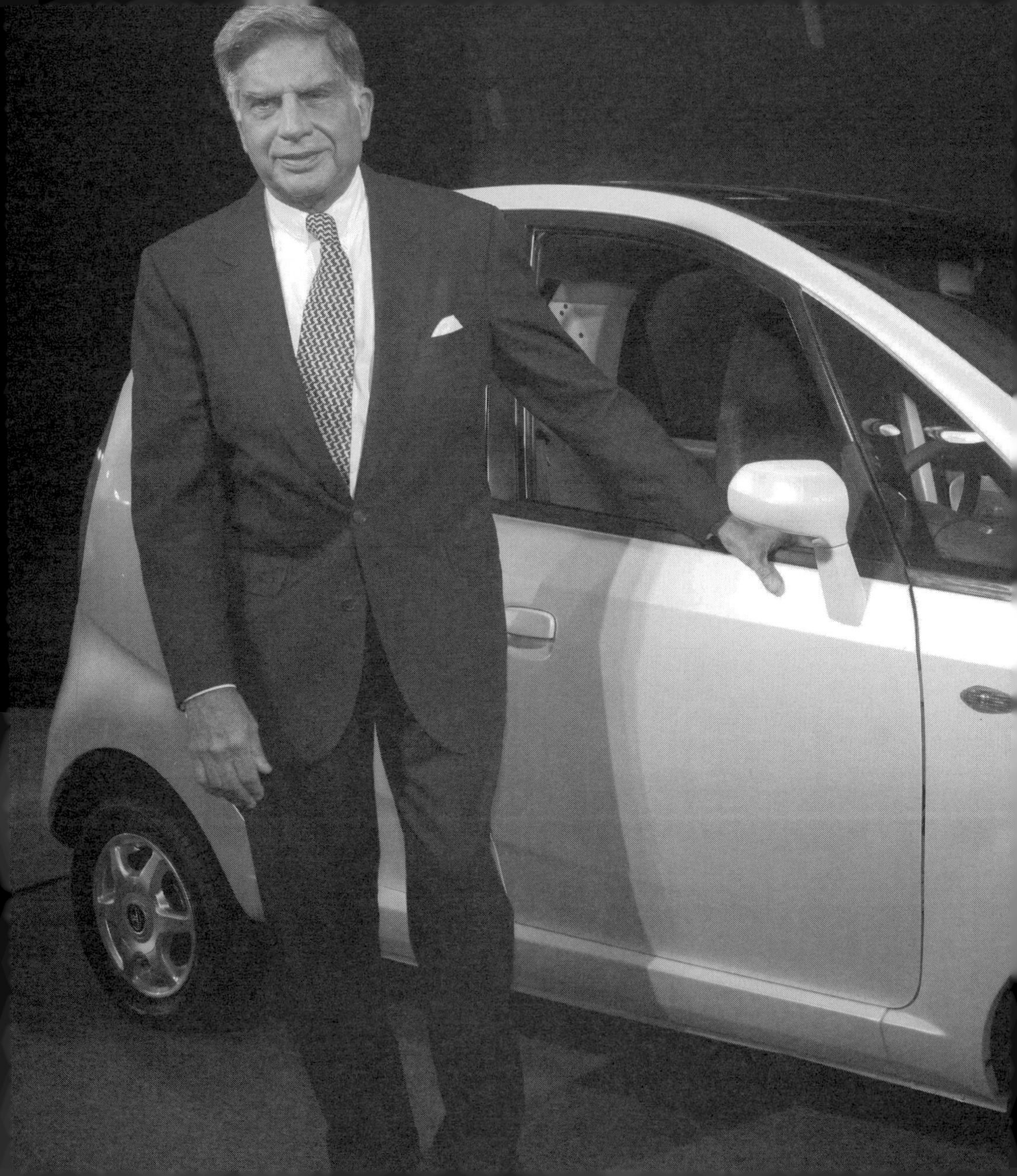

The Nano project has proven to everyone that if you really set yourself to doing something, you actually can do it.

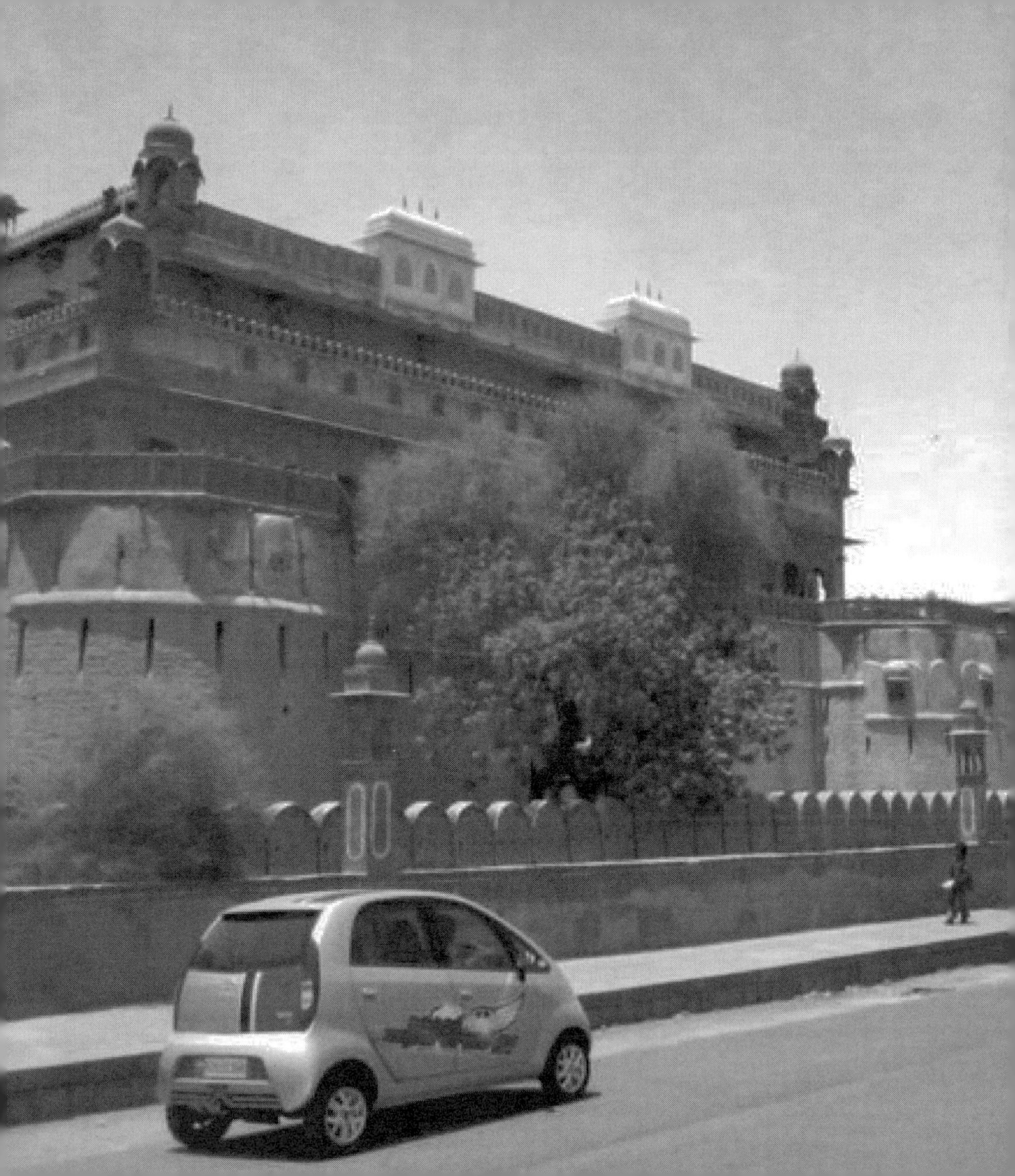

I have a view that the Nano can be marketed differently from how it is today. It can, with some evolution, be re-launched and made to serve the purpose for which it was intended. The Nano was meant to be an affordable car for the family, a vehicle that delivers outstanding value for money. Unfortunately, it has come to be perceived as a low-priced car and various stigmas have been attached to it. It has been marketed like other cars, but as a minimal automobile at a low price.

BRITAIN

&

JAGUAR LAND ROVER

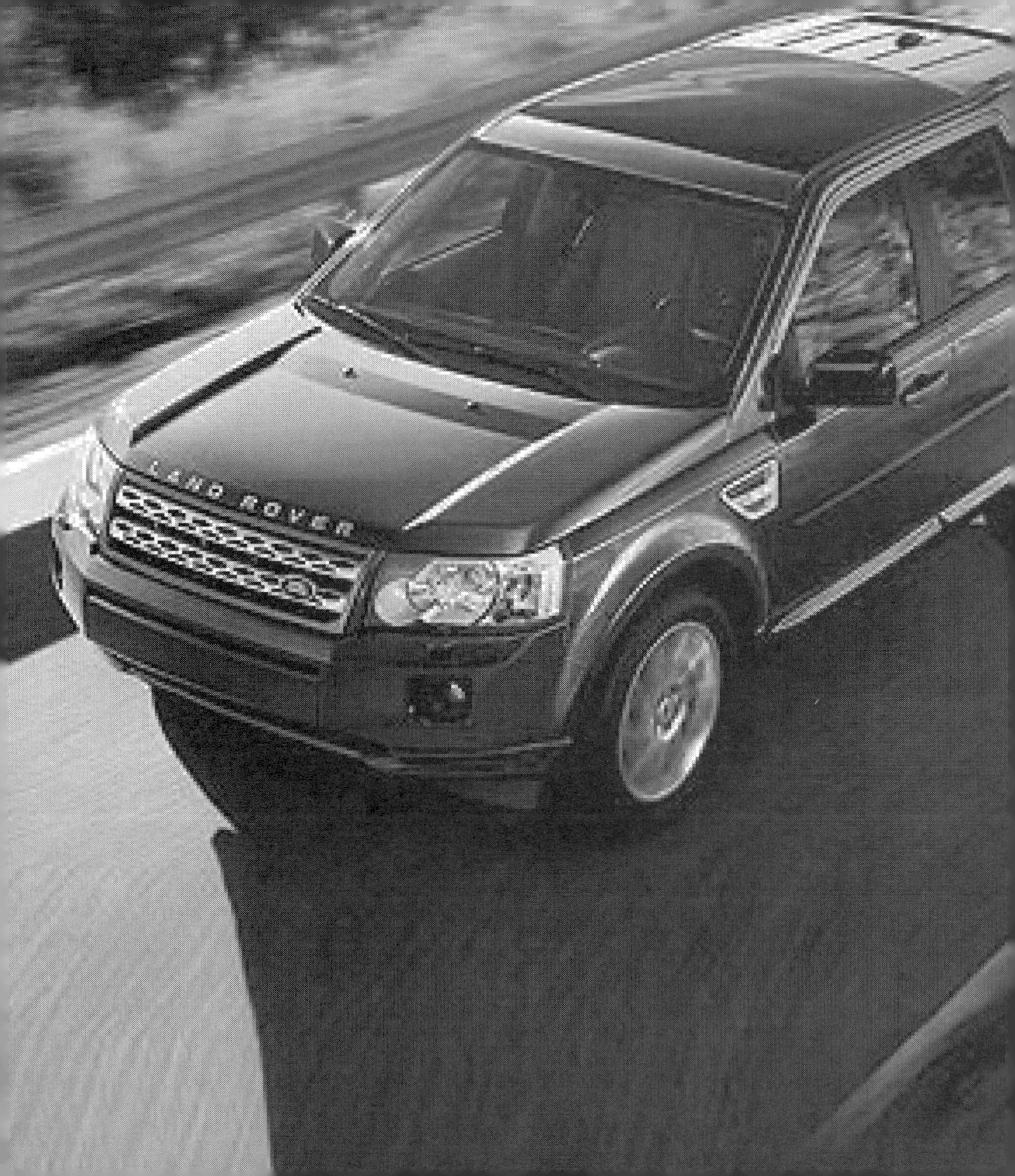
LAND ROVER

The Tata group has embarked on a journey of growth and geographical expansion and the acquisition of Jaguar Land Rover has put us in the international marketplace. It has made us sensitive to the volatility of those international markets and fuel prices.

I think the general change that I see in Jaguar Land Rover now is that everybody has enthusiasm about what they are doing, and confidence and faith in the direction the company is taking. We are not the magicians — they are the magicians.

HIS LEGACY

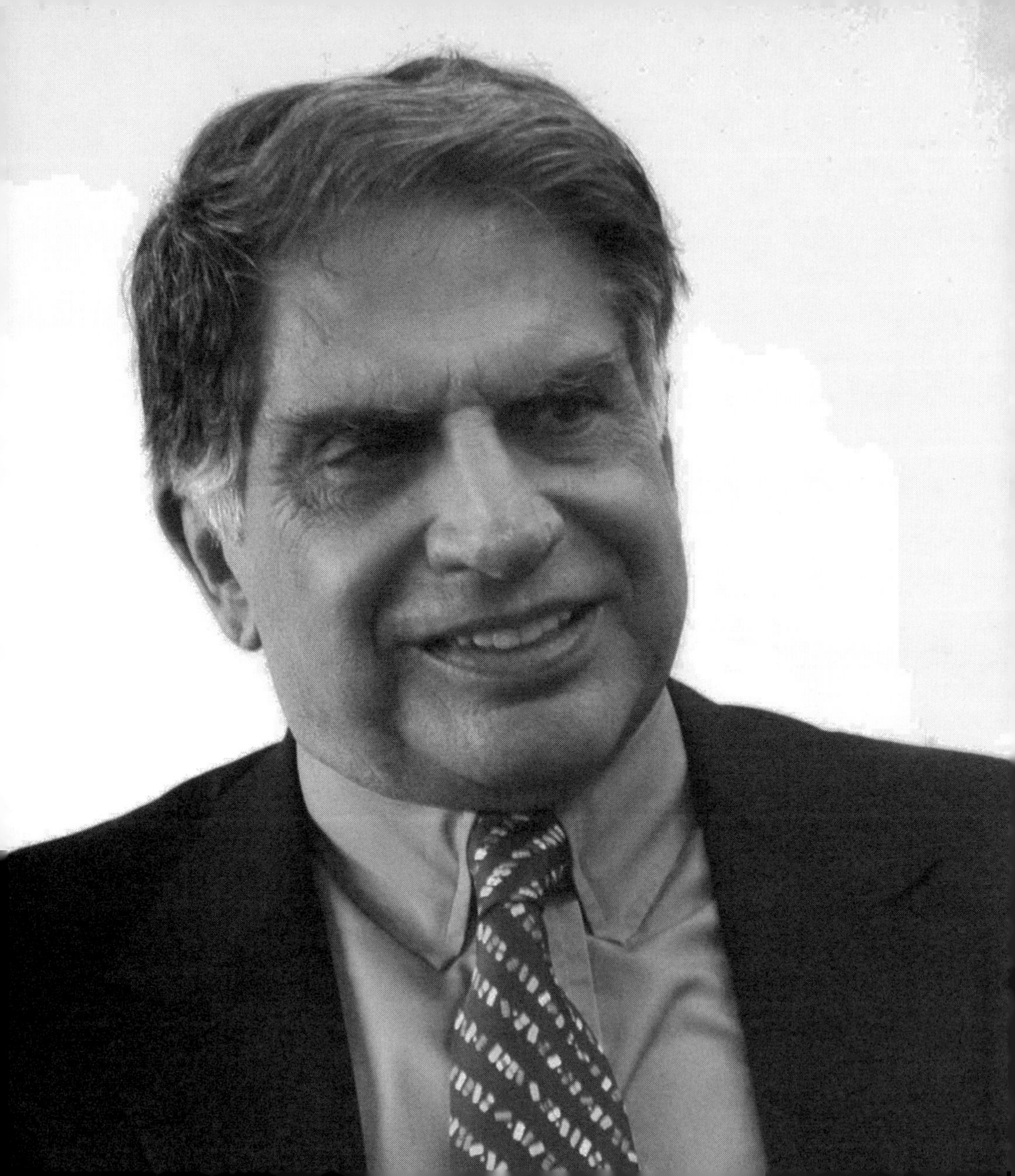

I have always tried to do the 'right' thing.

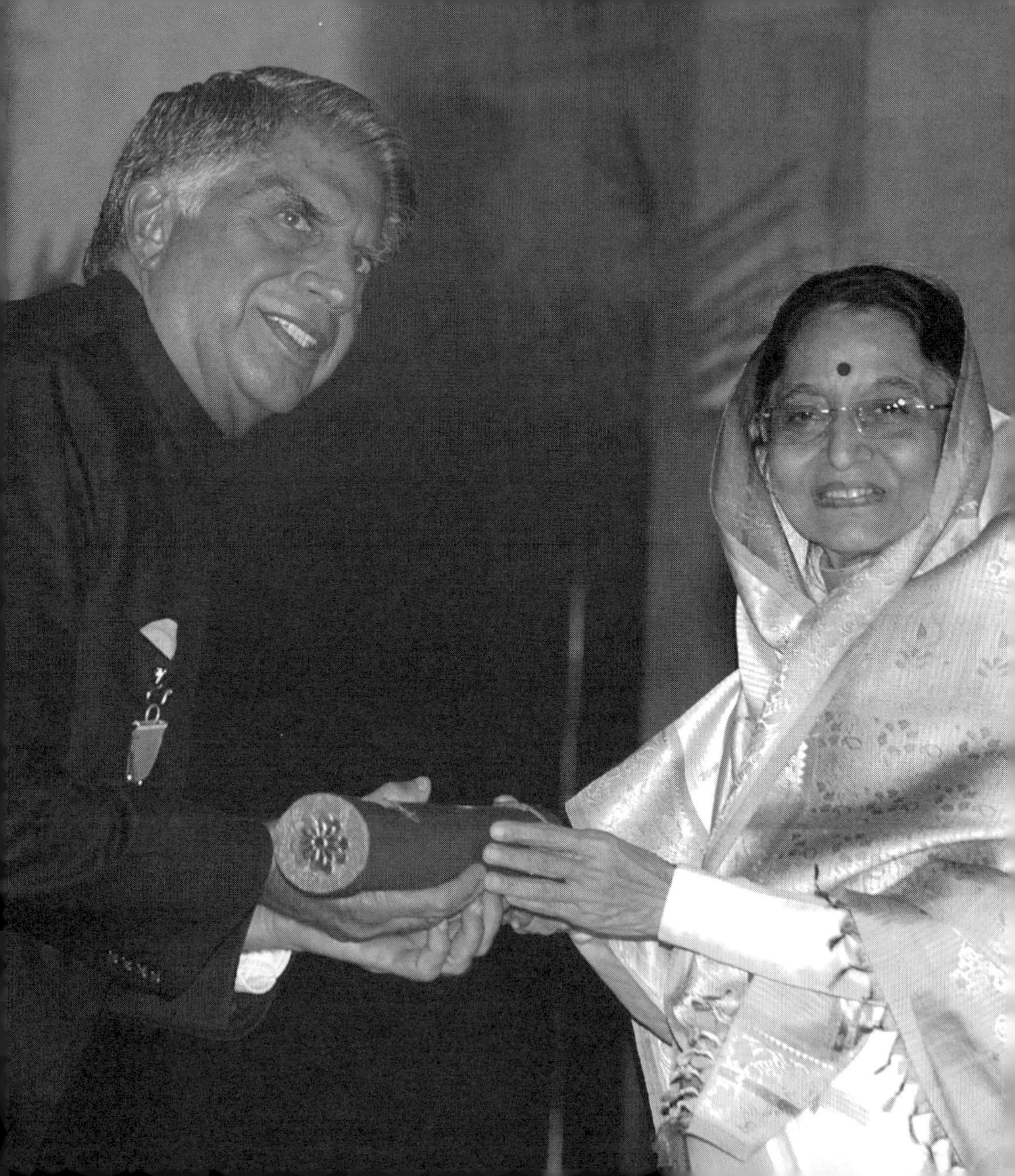

I would hope that people say I was able to lead the group with dignity...

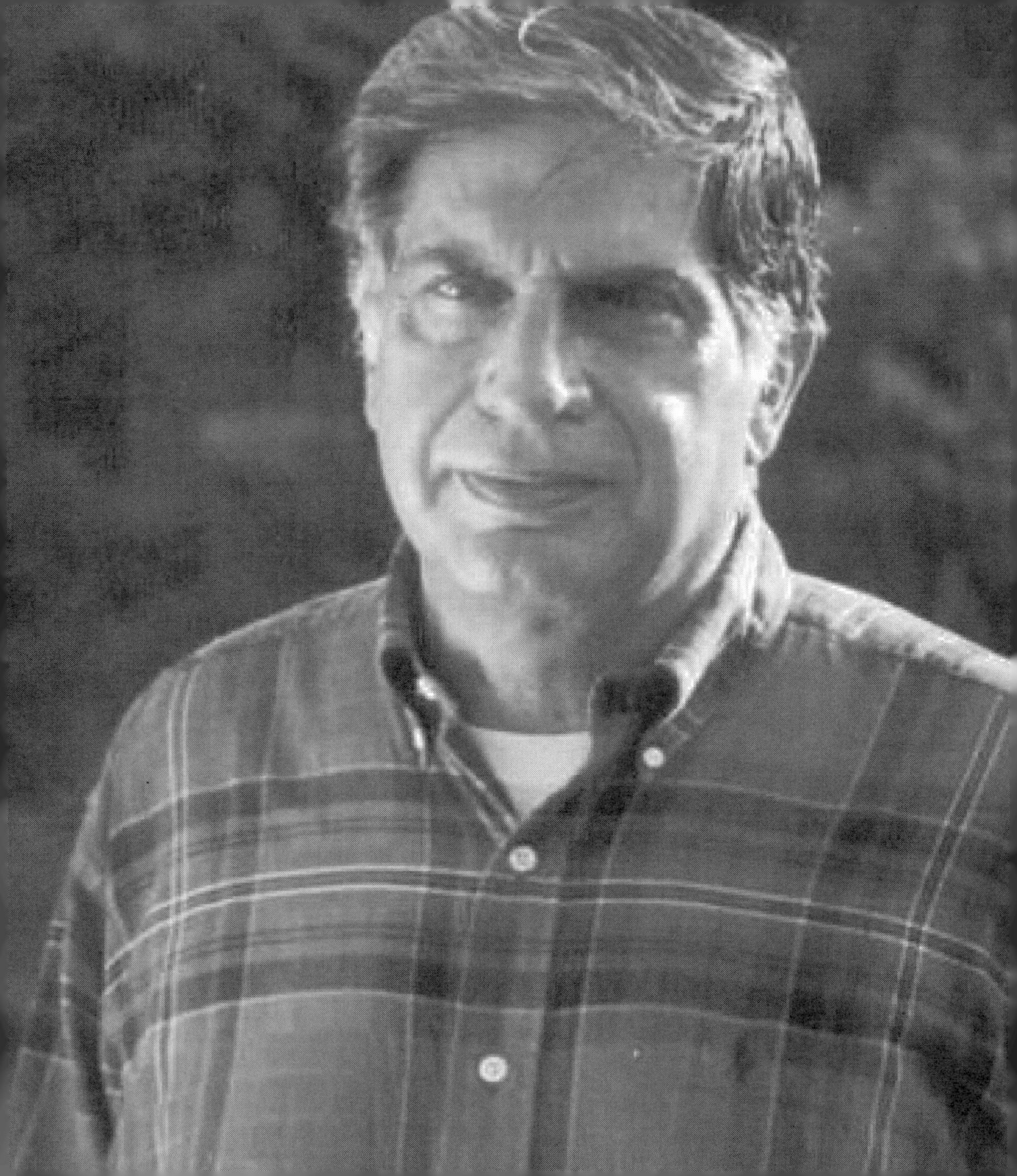

I would like to leave behind a sustainable set of companies that operate in an exemplary manner in terms of ethics and values, and build on what our ancestors left behind.

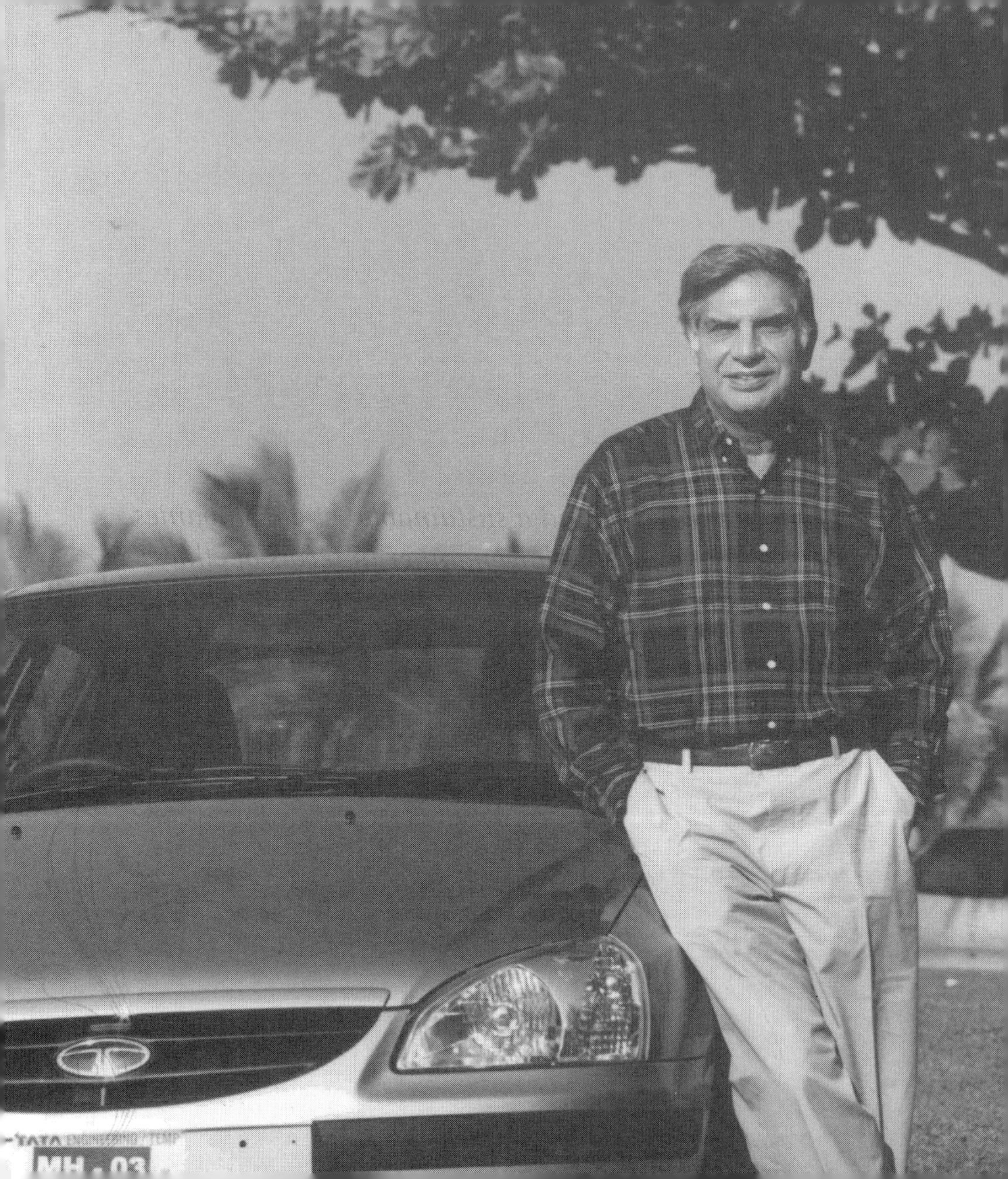
TATA
MH - 03

The legacy I leave behind – that which I am aware of, that which I can express – is that I myself have lived by the principles that I have desired for the group. I have led by example in that sense and I have devoted my life, as best I could, to the welfare of the group. I have endeavoured to do the best I could with the responsibilities I have had.

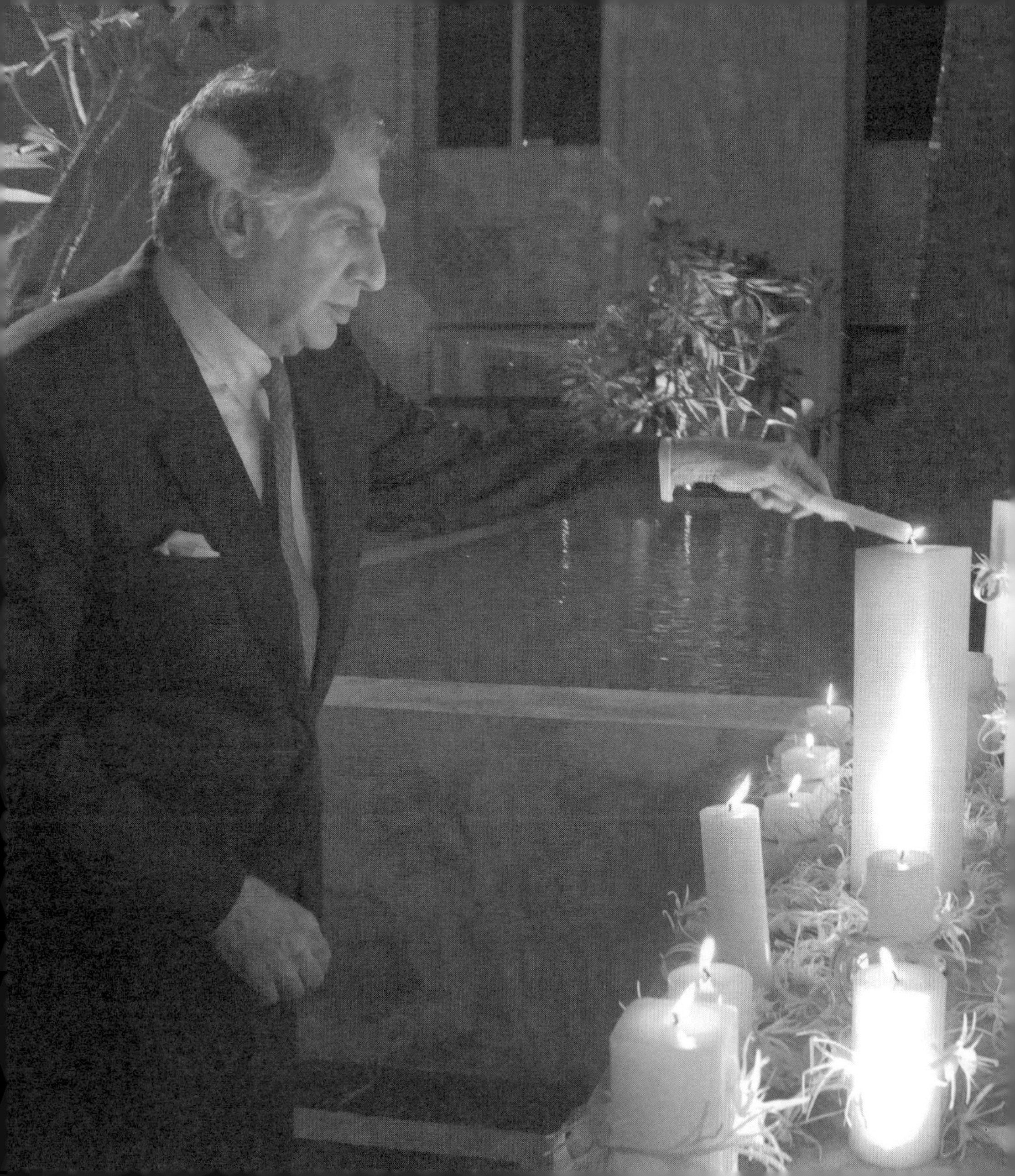

I do not know how history will judge me, but let me say that I've spent a lot of time and energy trying to transform the Tatas from a patriarchal concern into an institutional enterprise. It would, therefore, be a mark of failure on my part if it were perceived that Ratan Tata epitomises the group's success.

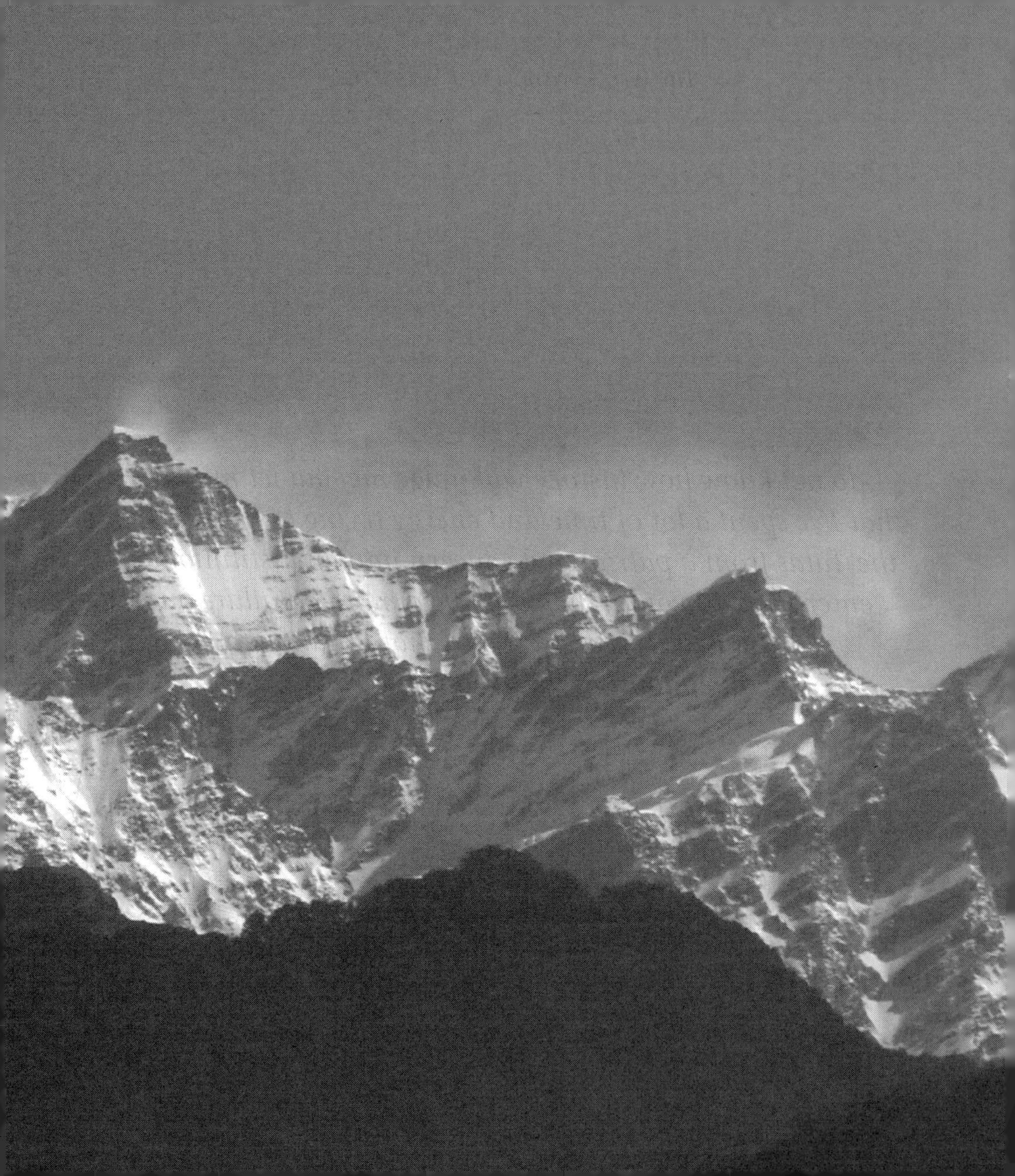

What I have done is establish growth mechanisms, play down individuals and play up the team that has made the companies what they are. I, for one, am not the kind who loves dwelling on the 'I'. If history remembers me at all, I hope it will be for this transformation.

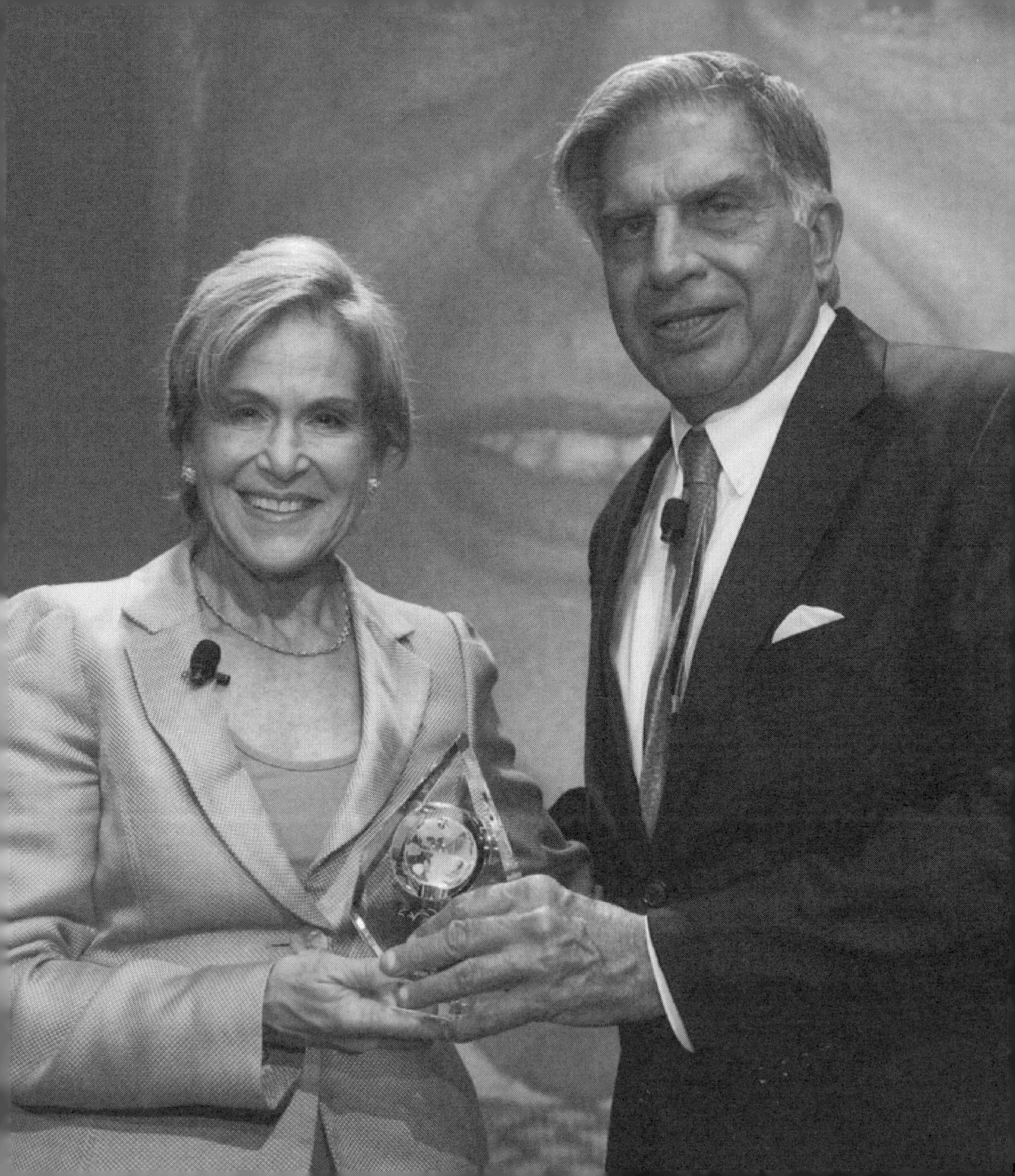

I would not consider myself to have been tremendously successful or as having failed tremendously. I would say I have been moderately successful.

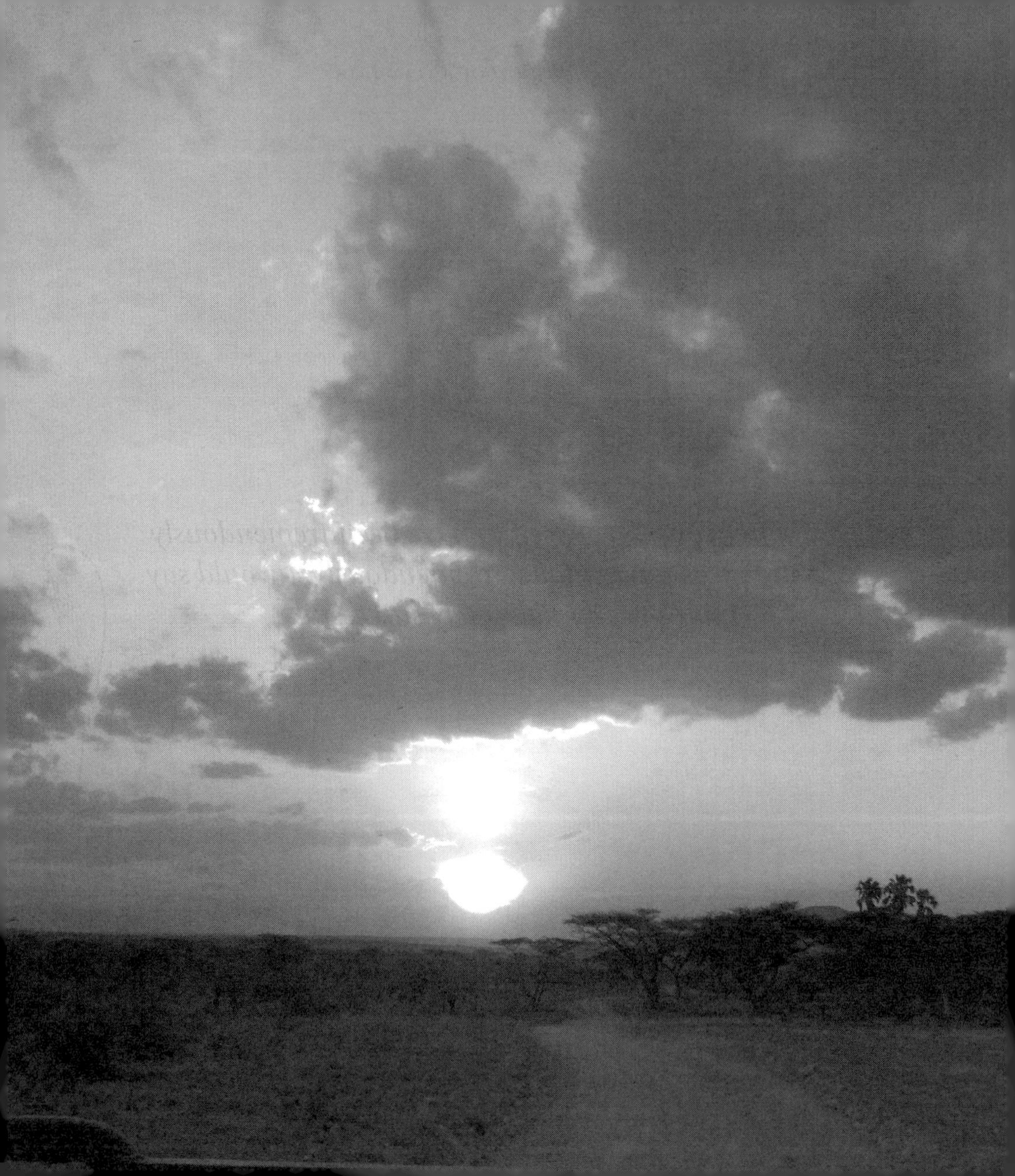

I don't want to have my shadow hanging over the group, a ghost walking the corridors.

(On the eve of his retirement)

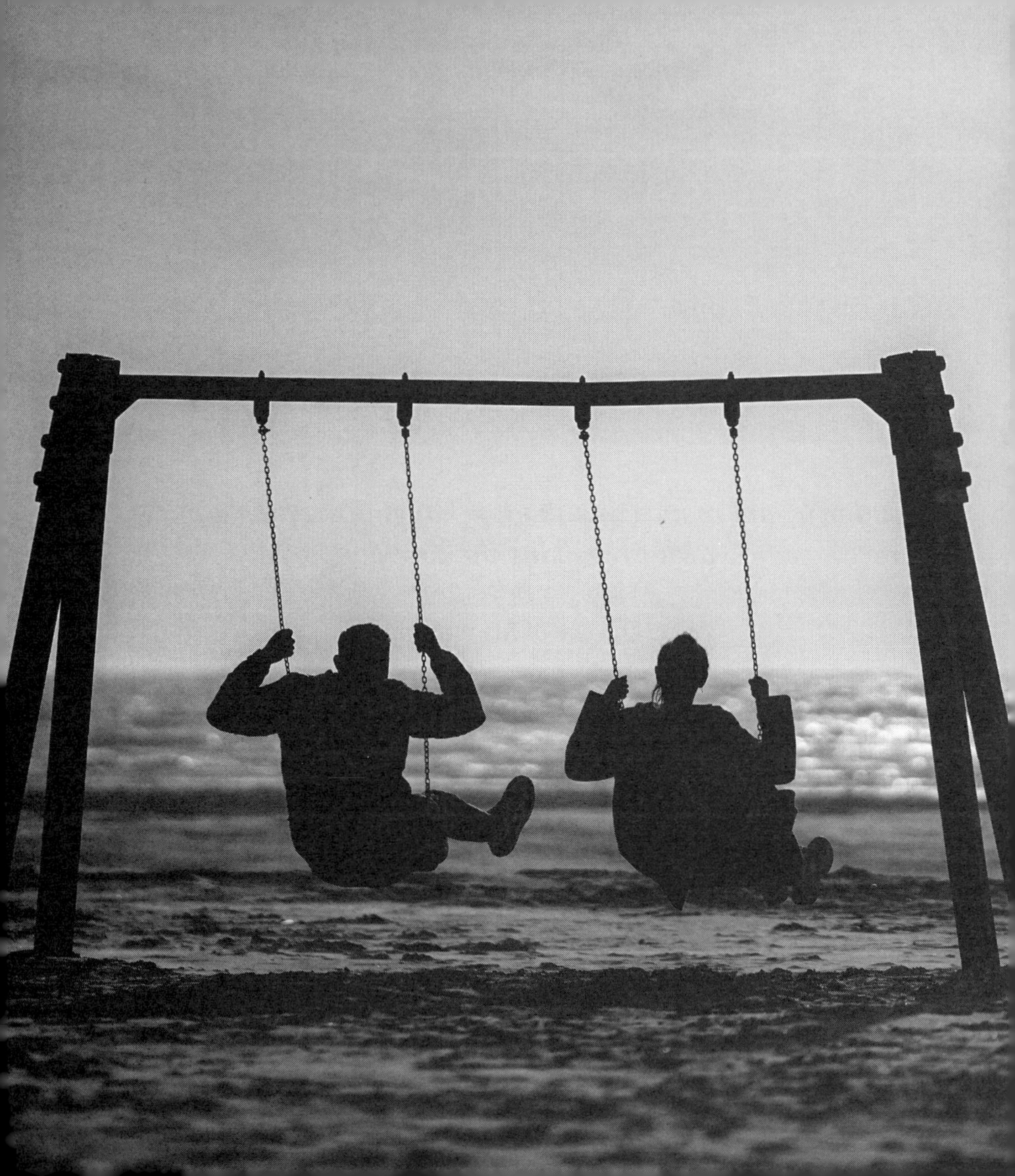

I don't believe in work-life balance.
I believe in work-life integration.
Make your work and life meaningful and fulfilling,
and they will complement each other.

DOING BUSINESS

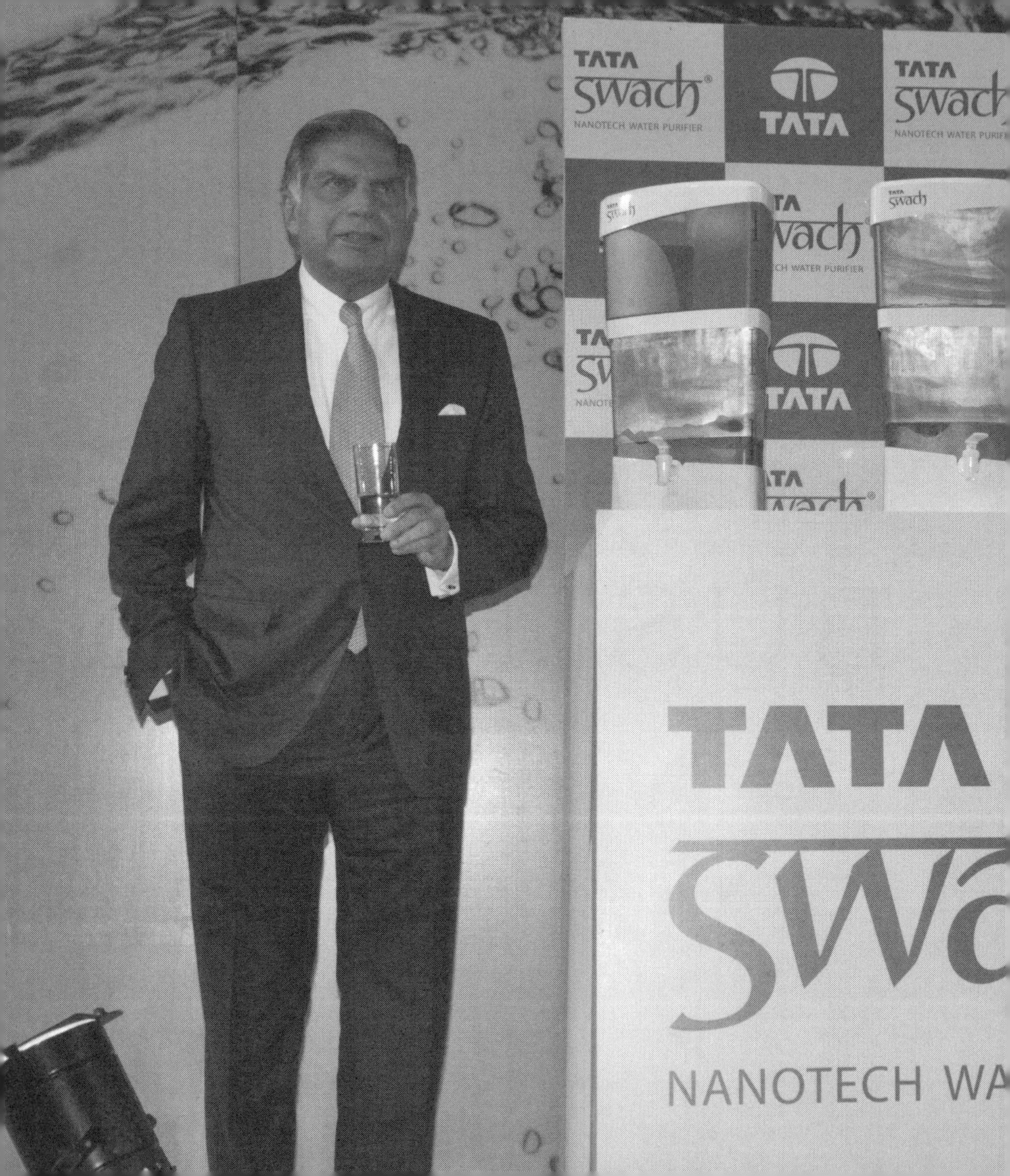
TATA
swach
NANOTECH WATER PURIFIER
TATA
TATA
swach
NANOTECH WATER PURIFIER
TATA
swach
NANOTECH WA

The strong live and the weak die. There is some bloodshed, and out of it emerges a much leaner industry, which tends to survive.

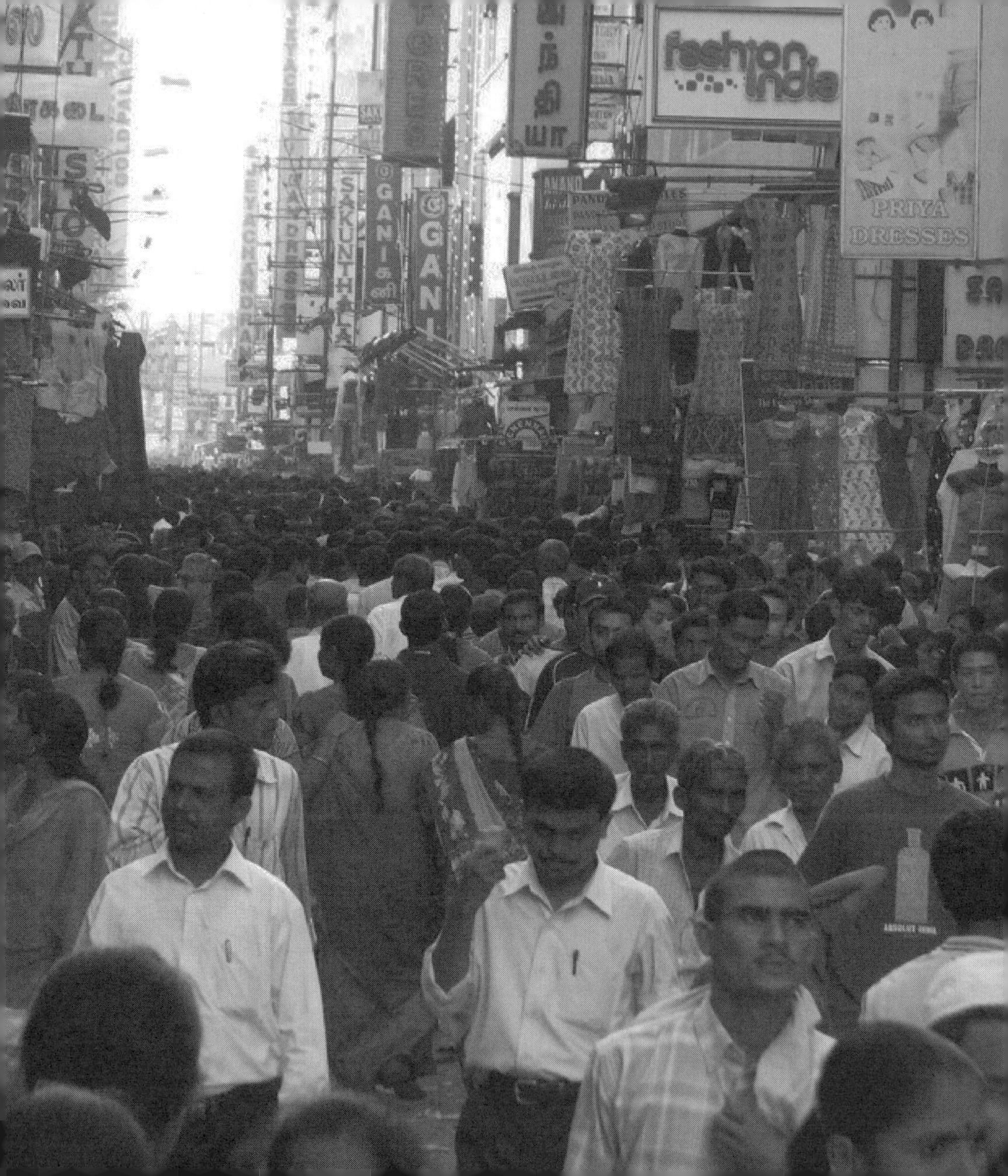
fashion india
PRIYA
DRESSES
GANI

We live in a highly competitive world – and we Indians have to struggle to catch up.

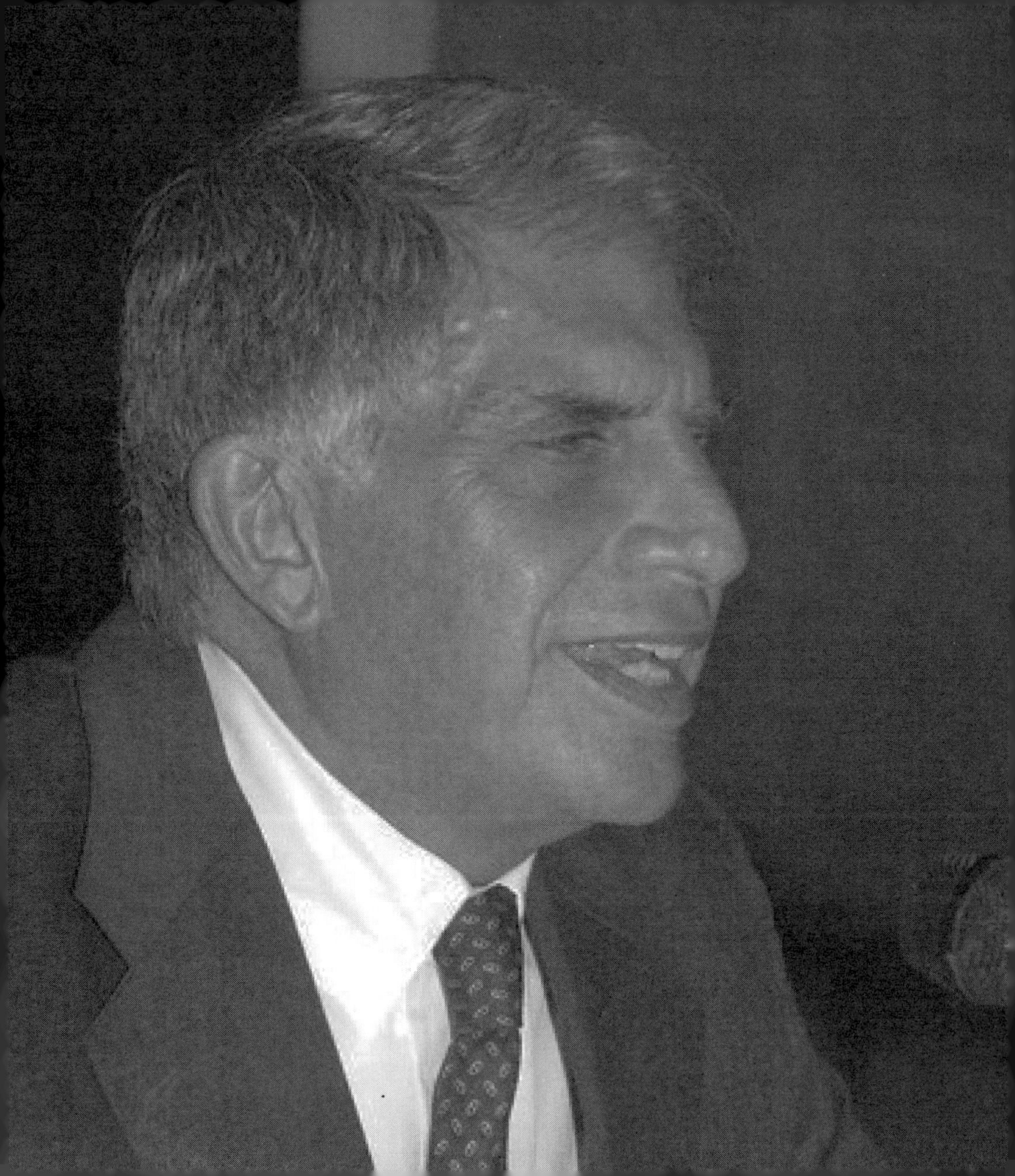

One of the weaknesses of Indian industry is that in many areas, like consumer goods, it is very fragmented. What is needed is a consortium of like companies in one industry, presenting a strong front to the multinationals.

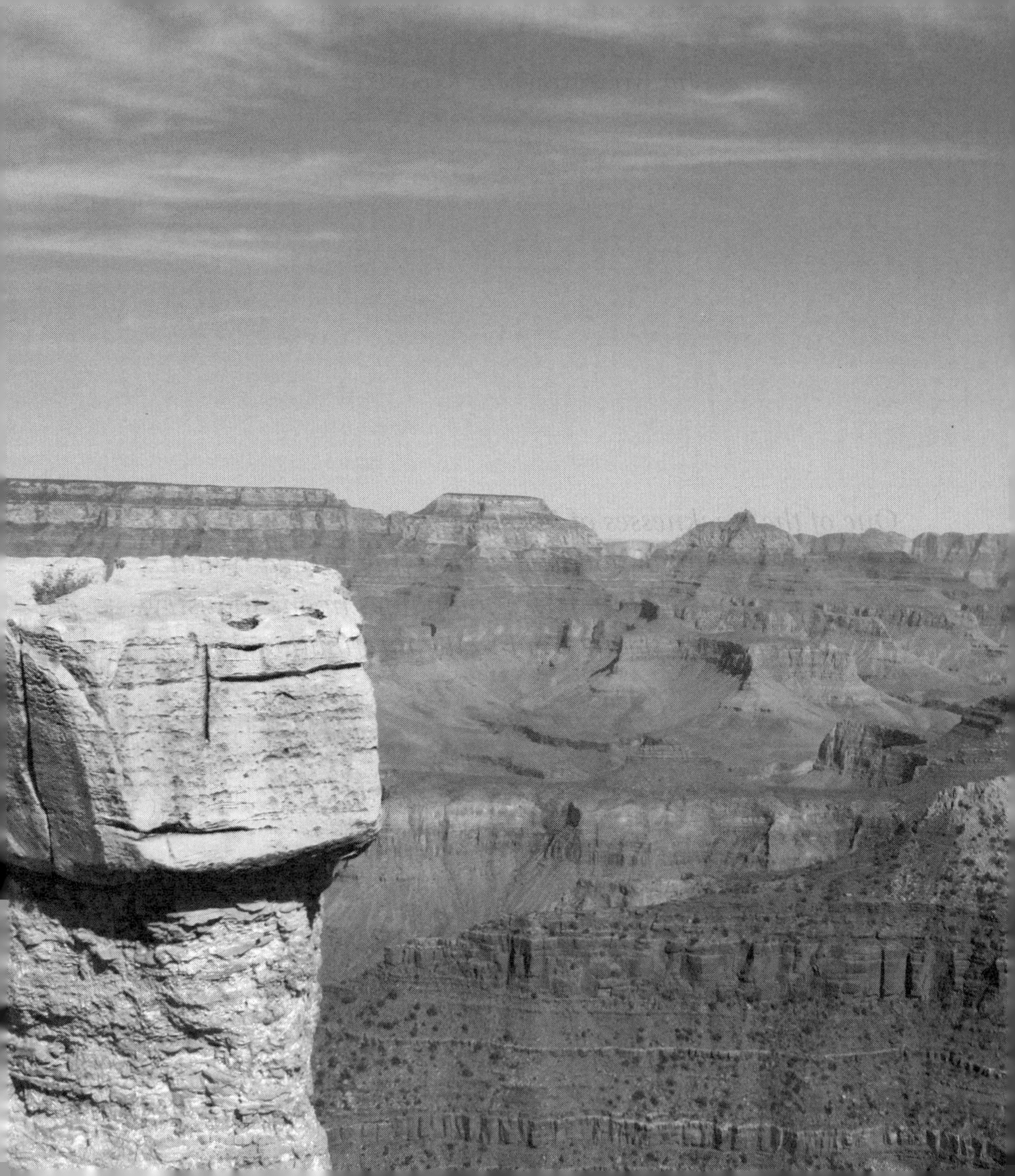

I've never believed protectionism will lead us anywhere. I think you can have certain specific rules for engaging with India, like, for example, not allowing mineral resources to be taken out of the country. But there is not a shred of doubt in my mind that when you open an economy you should do it in totality.

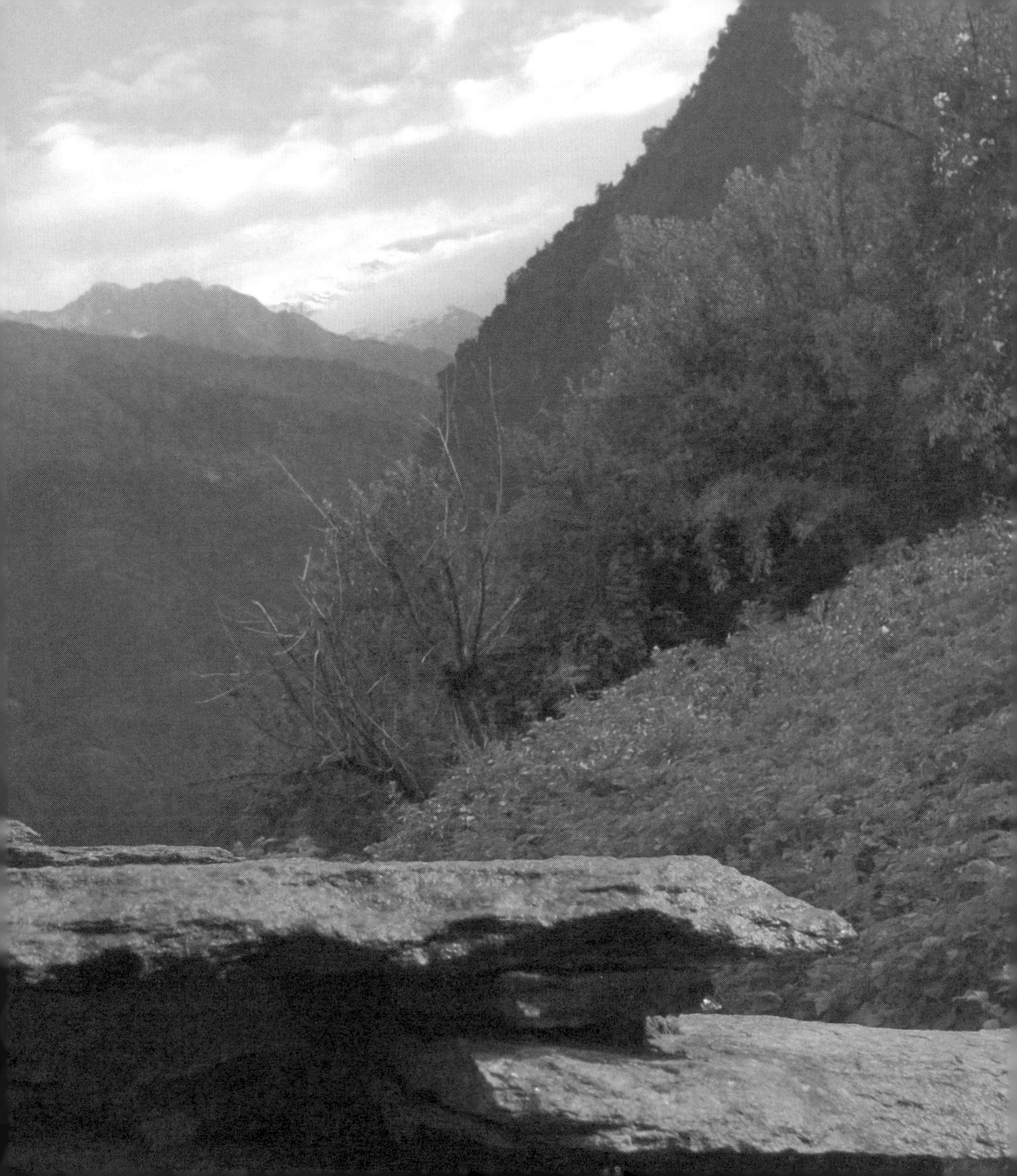

This fear of competition is something that one needs to break, because it is the single largest element that stands between the true potential of what India can give to the world and where it is today. It's a mistaken feeling that competition will kill Indian industry. In fact it will make Indian industry much more successful and much more innovative in terms of how it deals with its problems.

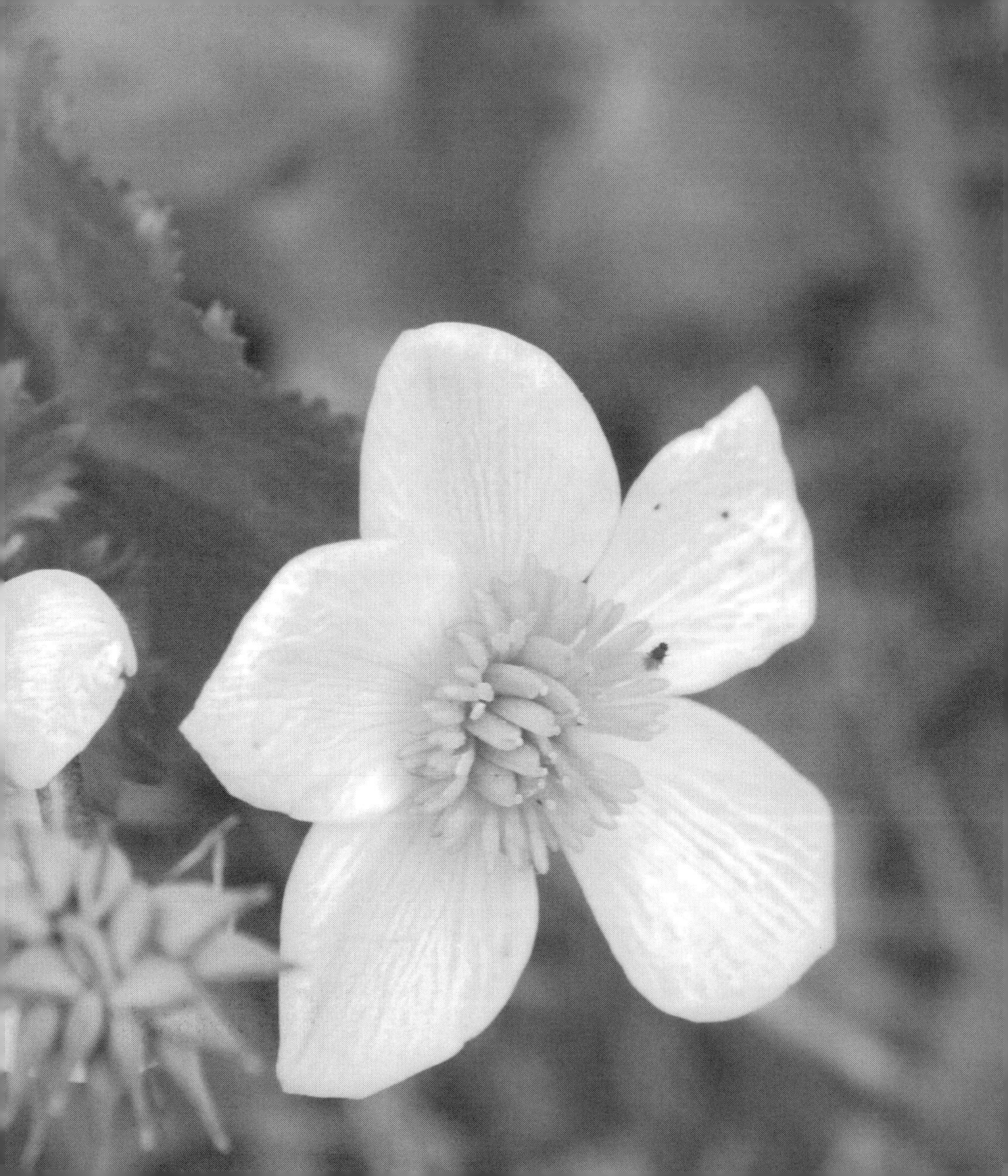

No group can hedge itself totally against a slowdown. The only hedge we can have is our operations in other geographies.

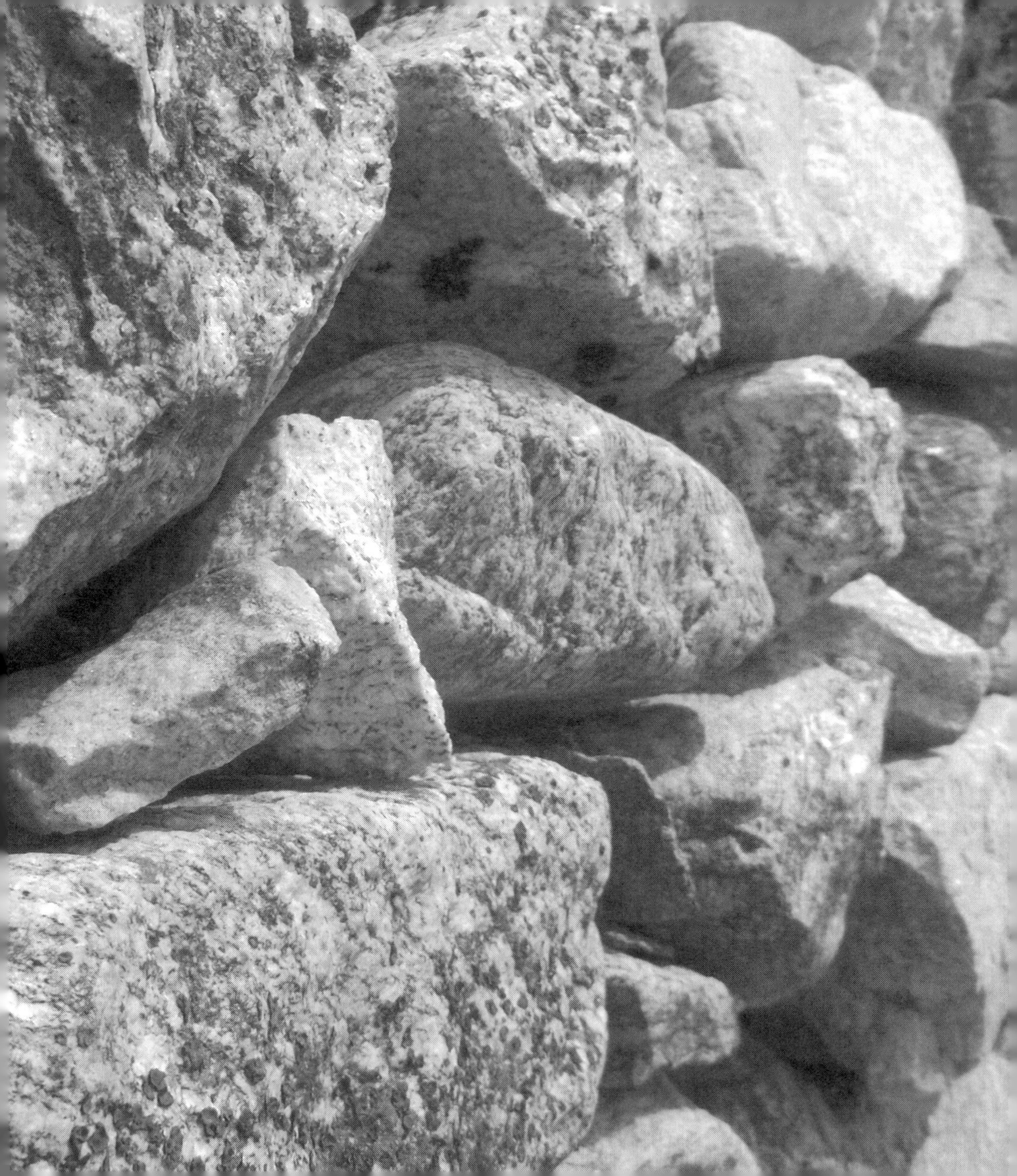

In my interactions with business leaders in India, there is this feeling that they are looking for cracks in your armour in order to pull you down. There is this tendency to look at the dark side of everybody and everything. Outside of India, in the business environment, there is genuine and much greater appreciation of the good that a person does and the success that he or she has achieved.

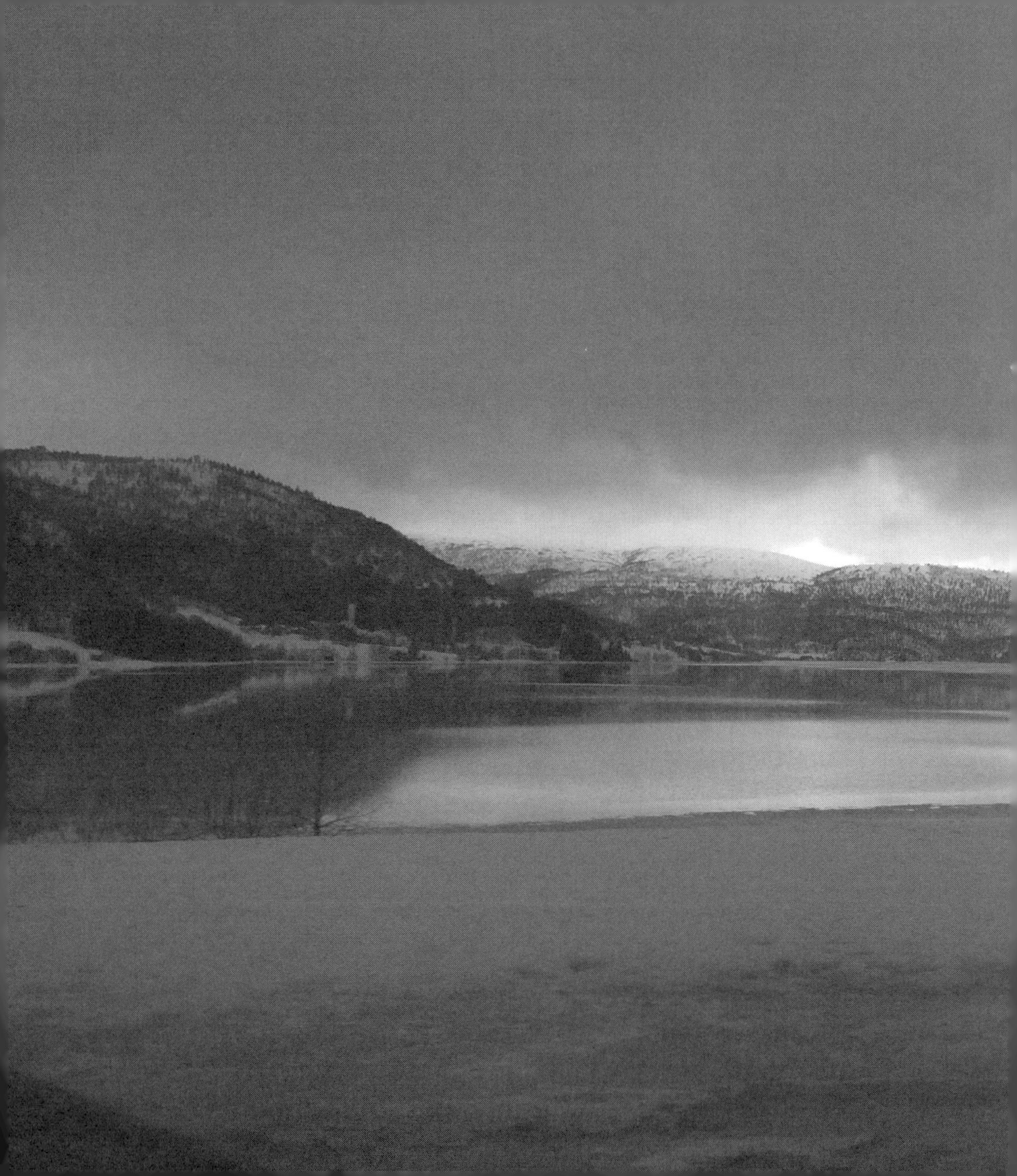

There have been occasions when I have been a risk-taker, perhaps more than some and less so than others; it's a question of where you view that from. I have never been a real gambler in the sense that some successful businessmen are.

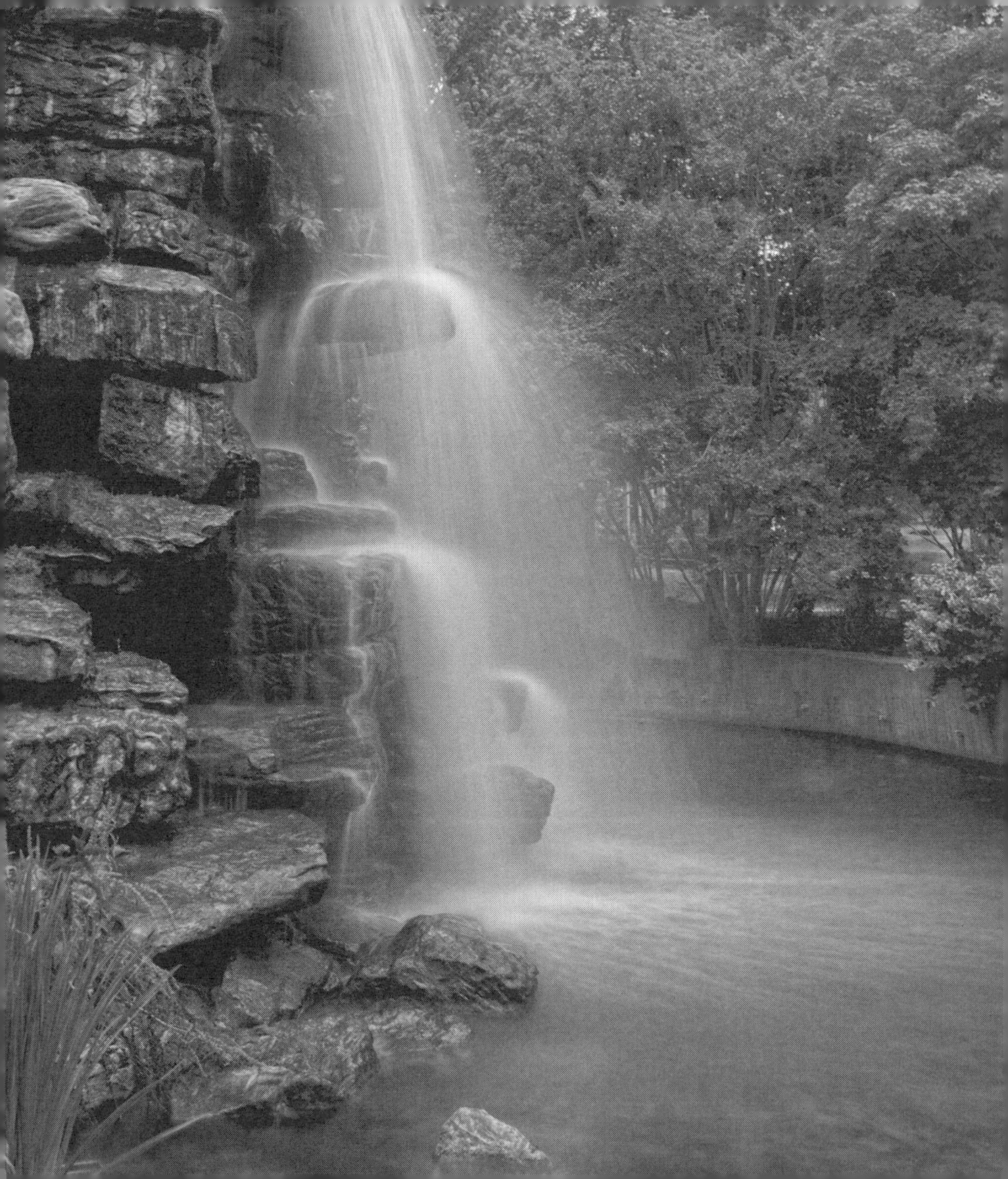

*I think risk is a necessary part of business philosophy.
I view risk as an ability to be where no one has been before.
I view risk to be an issue of thinking big.*

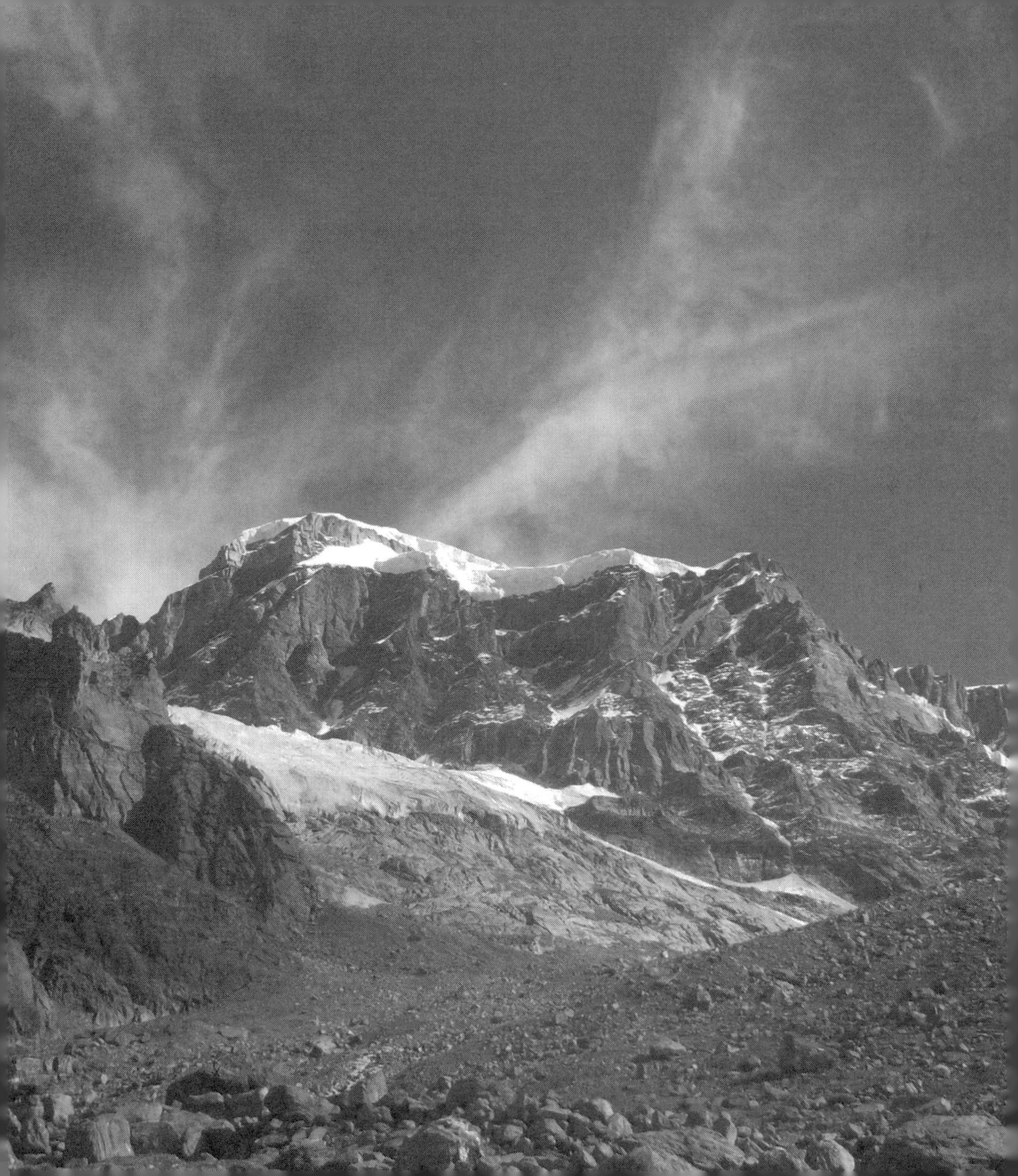

You can be risk-averse and take no risks, in which case you will have a certain trajectory in terms of your growth. Or you can, while being prudent, take greater risk in order to grow faster.

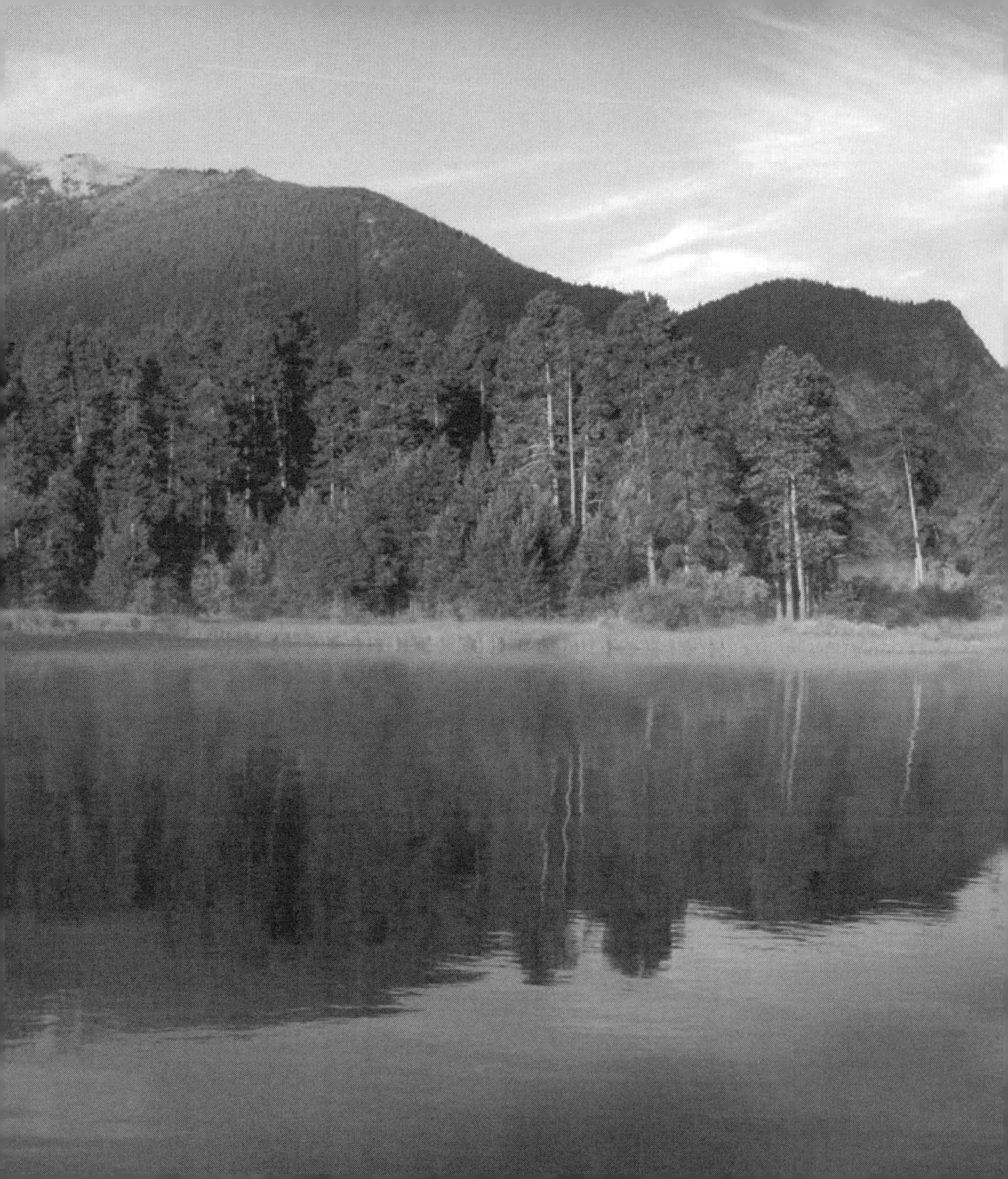

Barriers to innovation are usually in the mind.

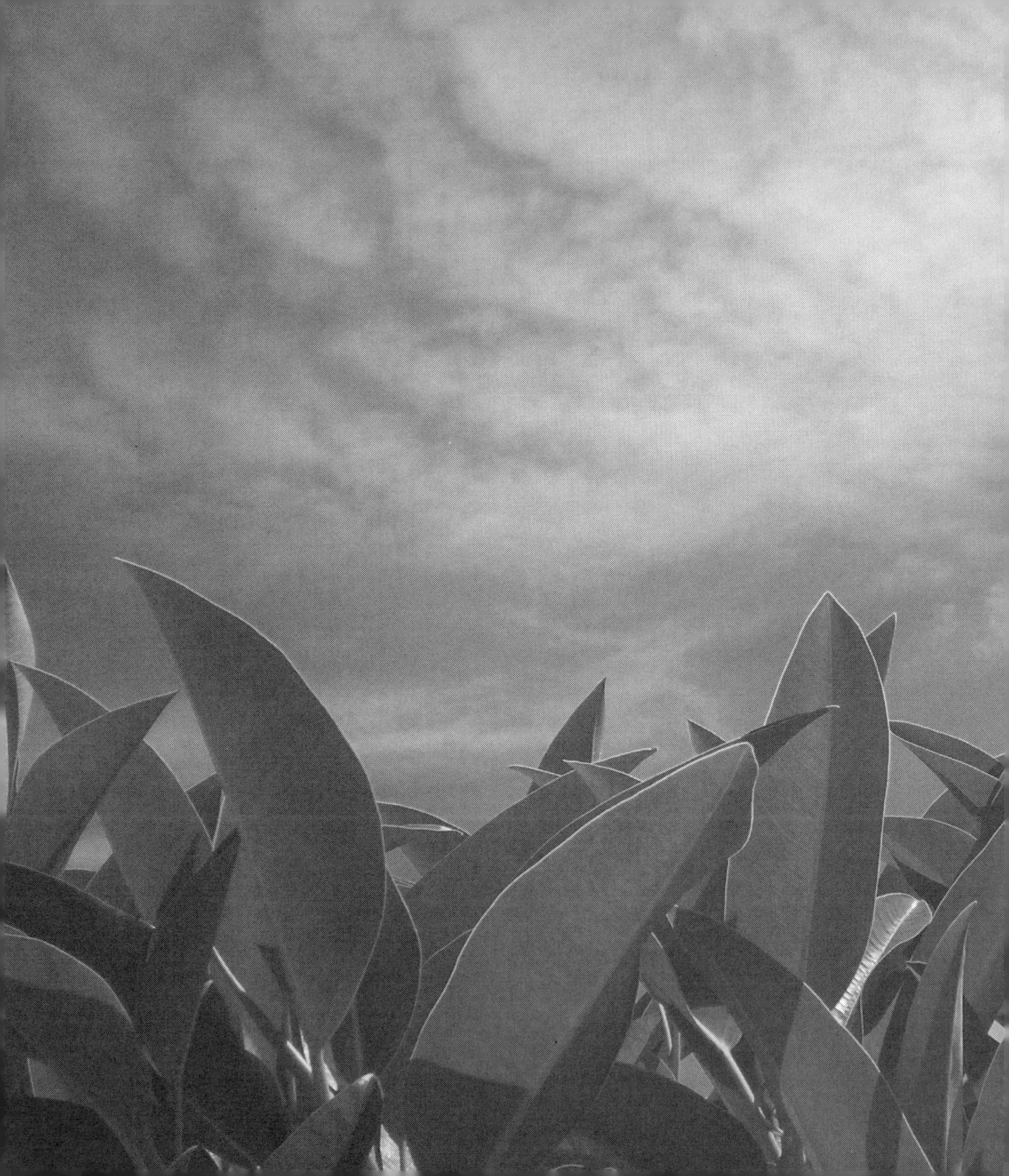

What worries me is that the threshold of acceptability, or the line between acceptability and non-acceptability in terms of values, business ethics, etc., is blurring.

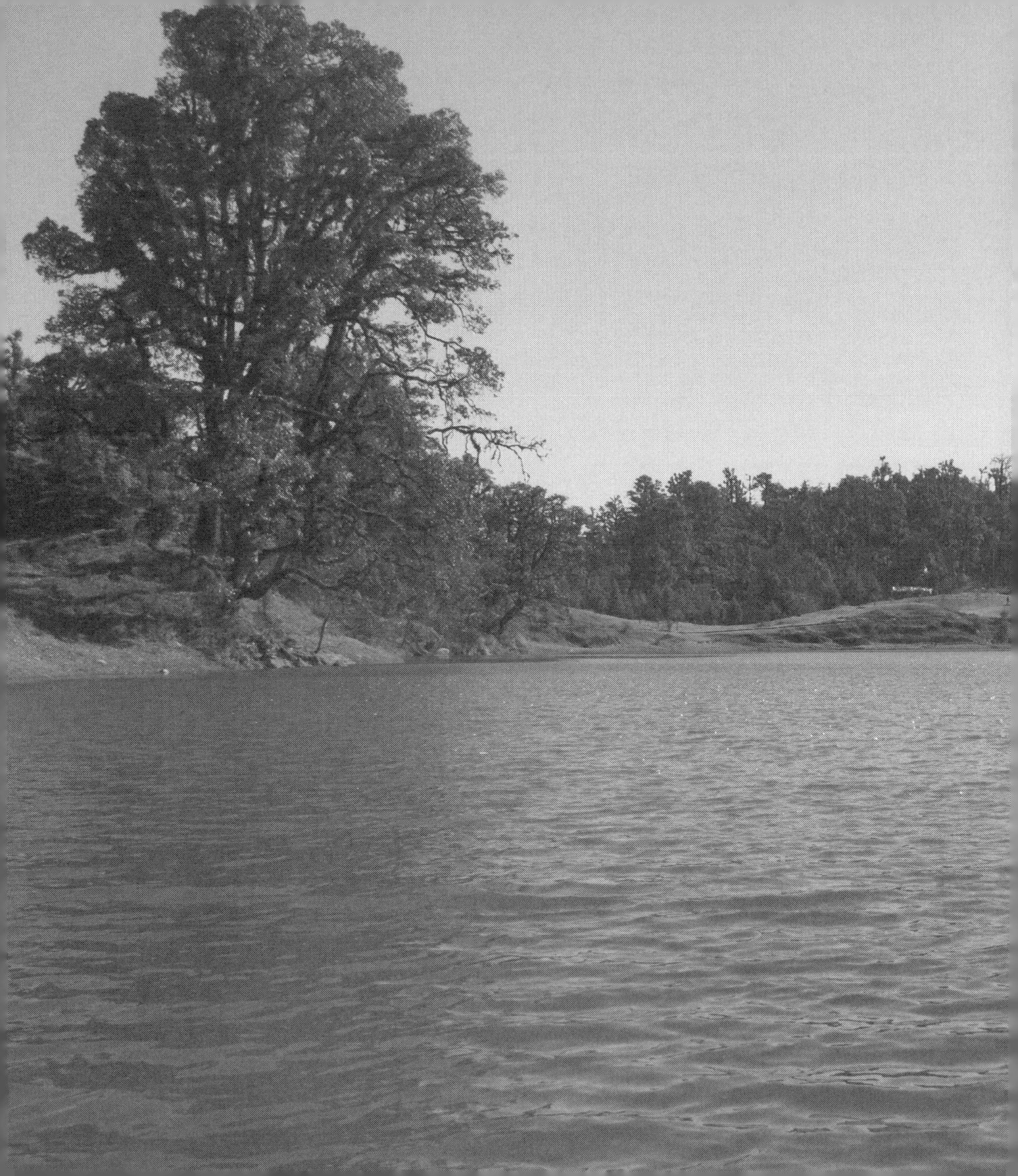

As a nation we seem to be following, more and more, a divergence towards a breakdown in the fabric of values and principles and ethics.

BEYOND BUSINESS

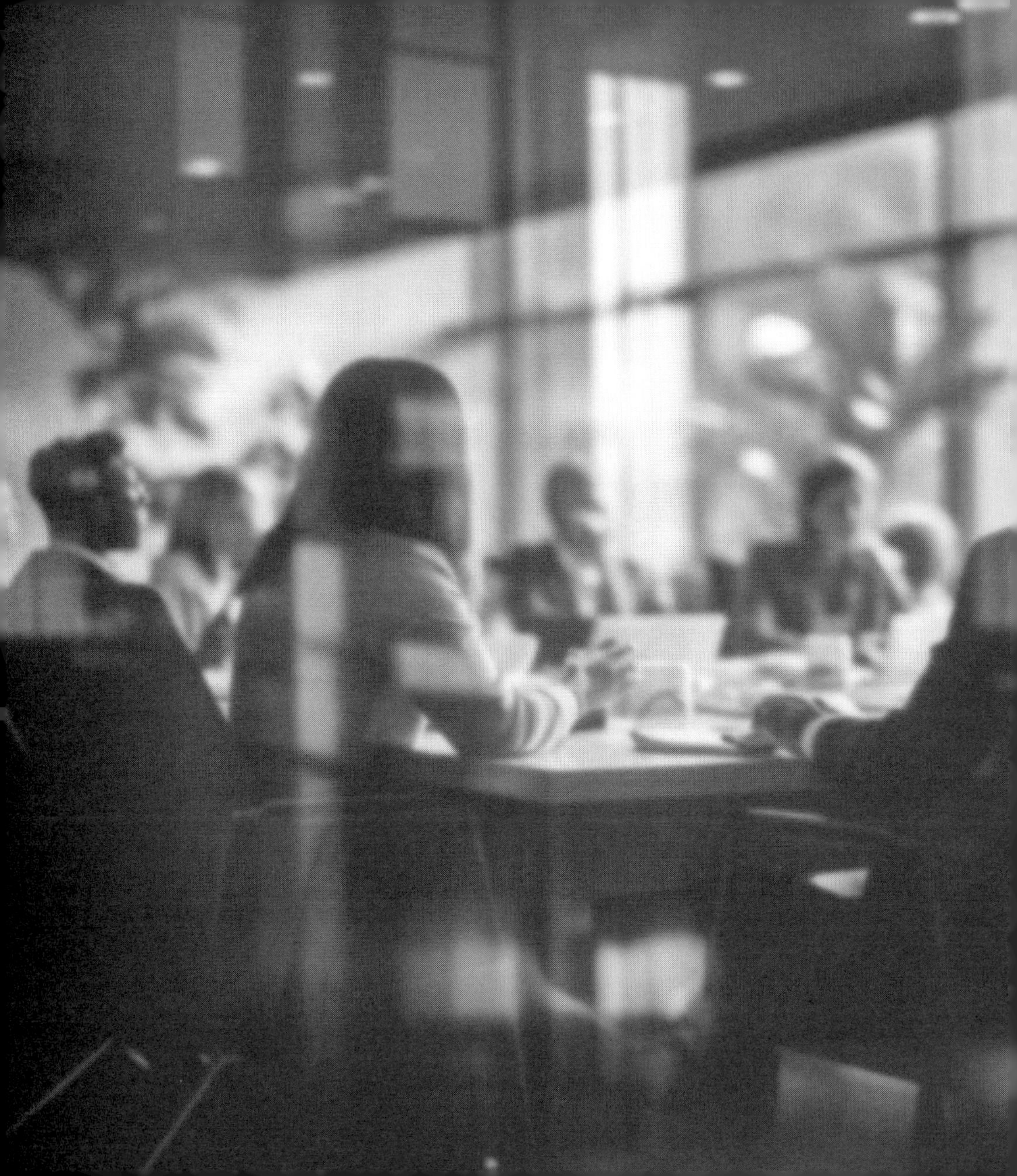

The best leaders are those most interested in surrounding themselves with assistants and associates smarter than they are.

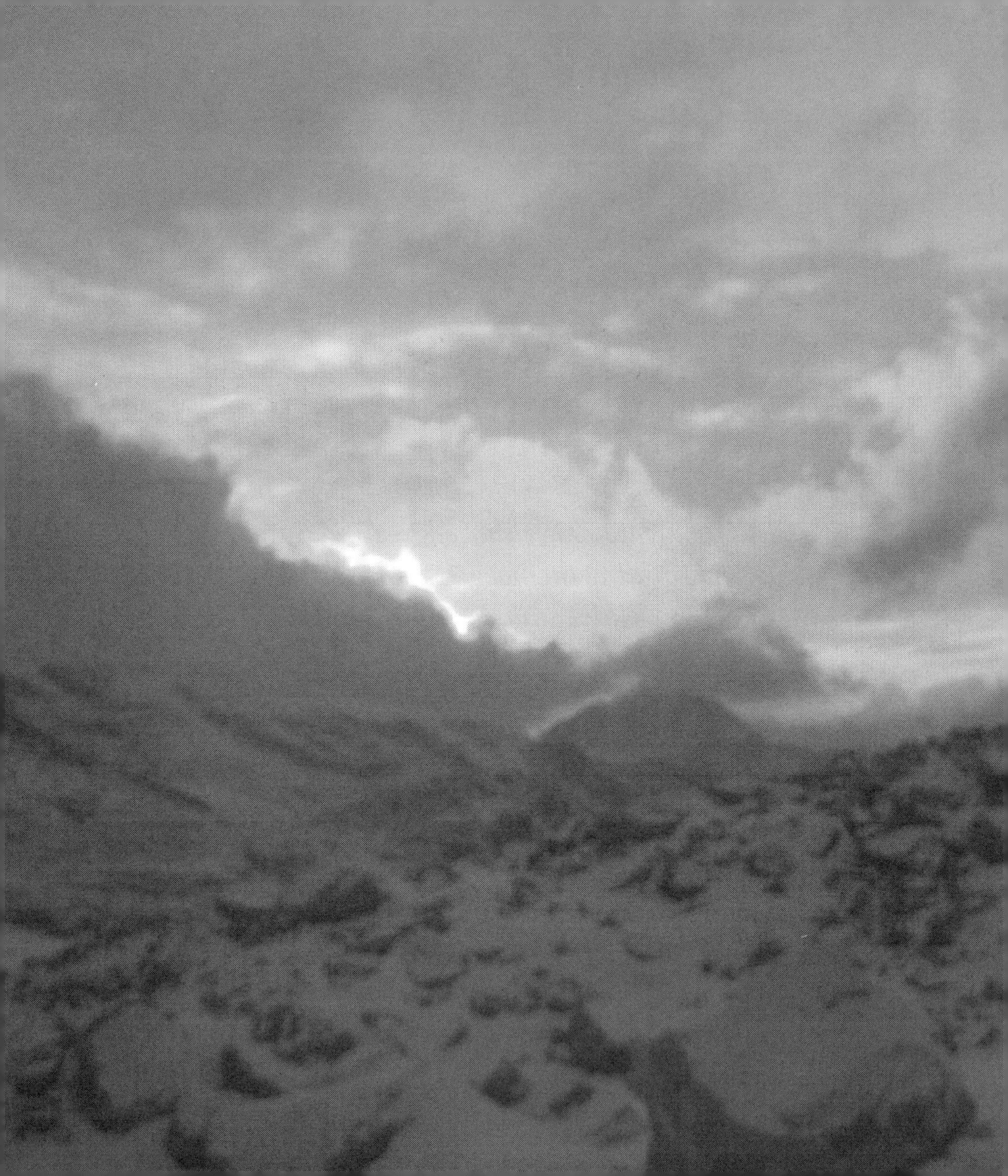

Businesses need to go beyond the interests of their companies to the communities they serve.

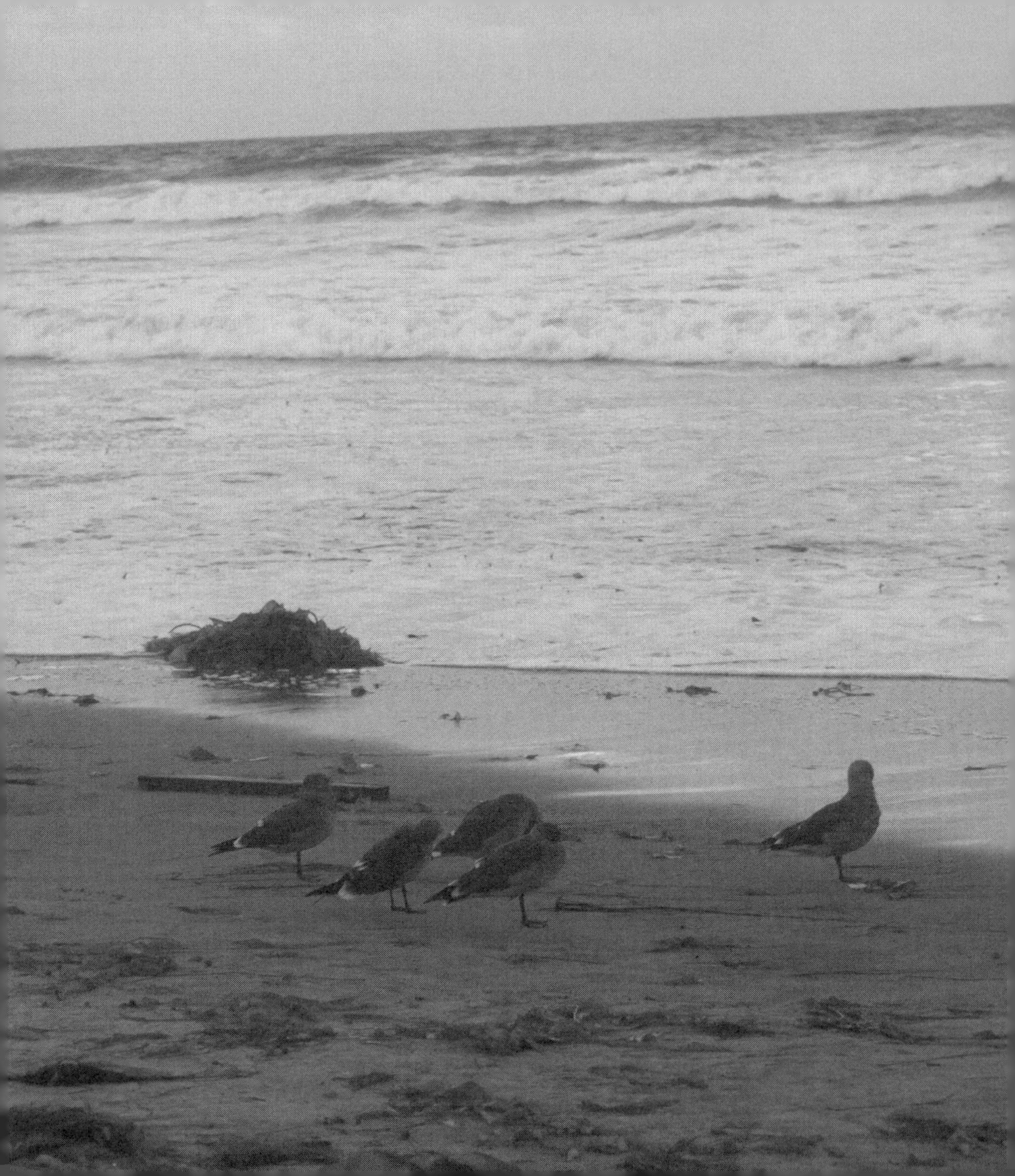

Businesses are under greater pressure than ever to generate profits, but this should never be at the expense of the environment. Companies have to be sensitive about sustainability, about issues such as pollution and the terrible consequences of carelessness or, worse, callousness.

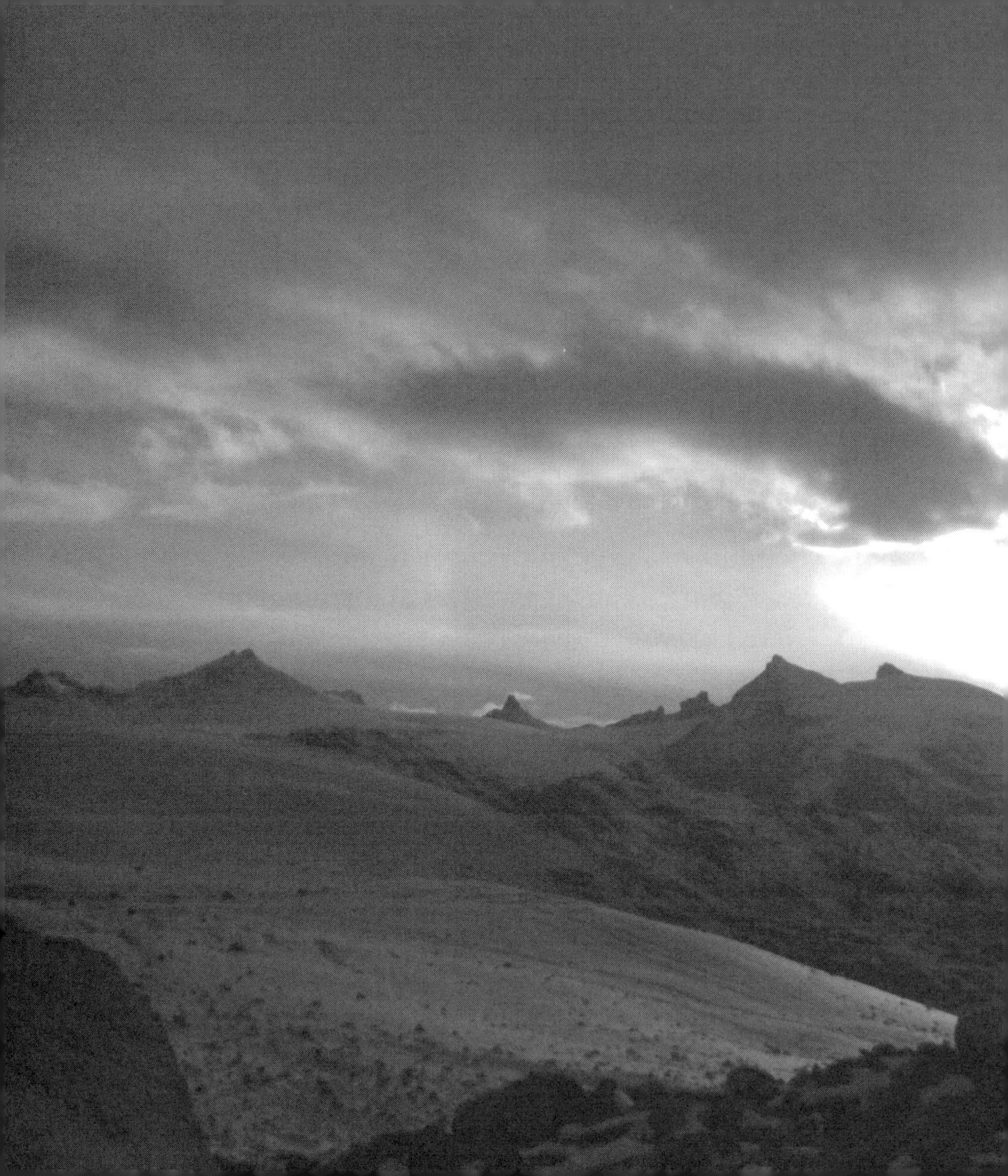

I believe that we, that is, Indian industry, should have the responsibility of doing something for the traditionally deprived, but quotas are not an answer. What is needed is to give people an equal opportunity, which they do not have today. And I think that equal opportunity will not come from quotas; it will come from having more primary schools for them, perhaps finding solutions that will enable their families to send them to school, instead of leaving them in a situation in which they have to pull them out of school to send them to work. I believe that equal opportunity will come from creating vocational training for them so that they can master a trade.

Industry needs to be concerned with stopping the flow of citizens to the urban areas and creating livelihoods in the rural areas for them. They need to understand that they have a responsibility that goes beyond just making their products and producing a good bottom line. They have a responsibility that covers the 60-odd per cent of the population that is not industrialised and that is in the rural community.

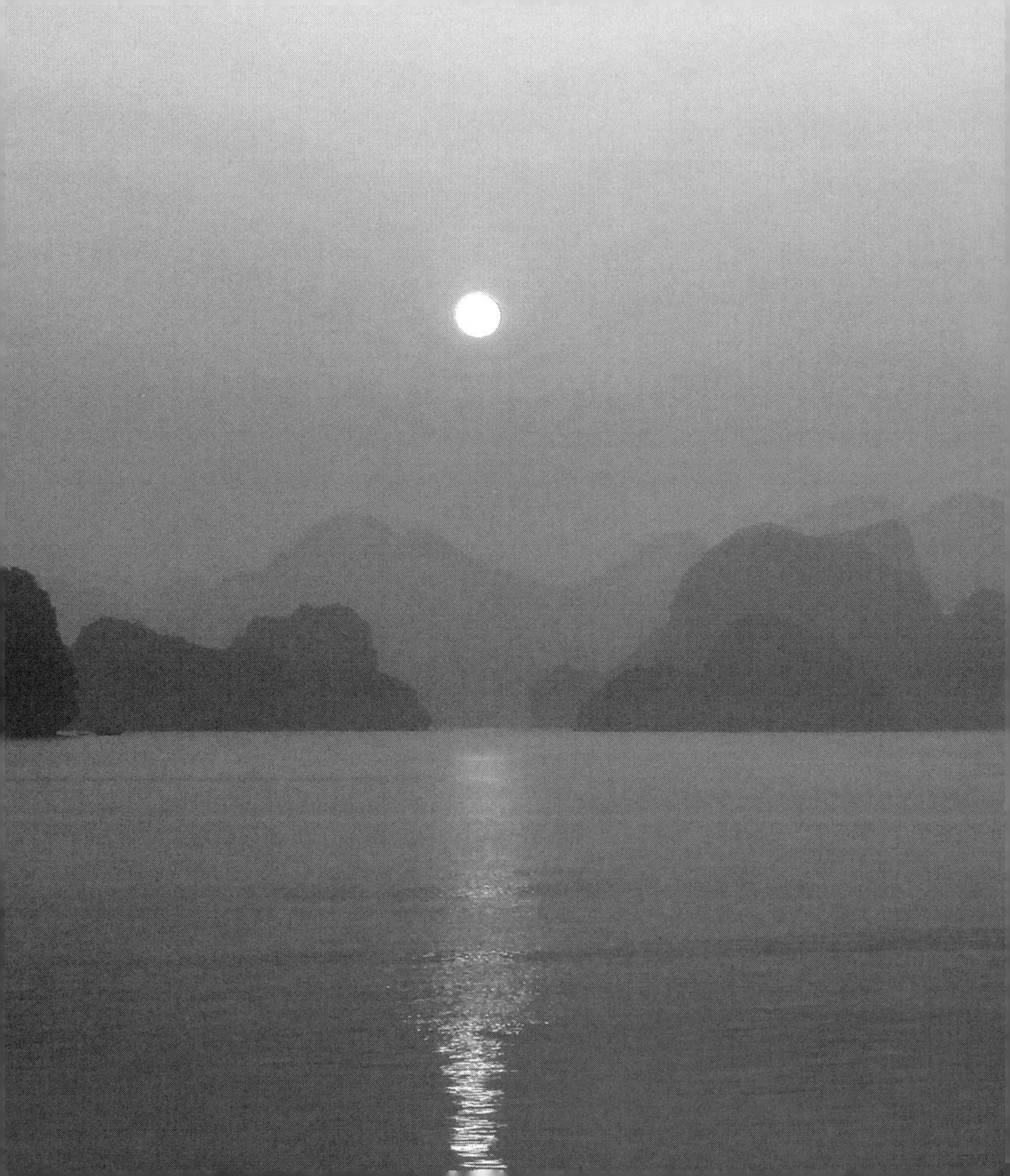

Some foreign investors accuse us of being unfair to shareholders by using our resources for community development. Yes, this is money that could have made for dividend payouts, but it also is money that's uplifting and improving the quality of life of people in the rural areas where we operate and work. We owe them that.

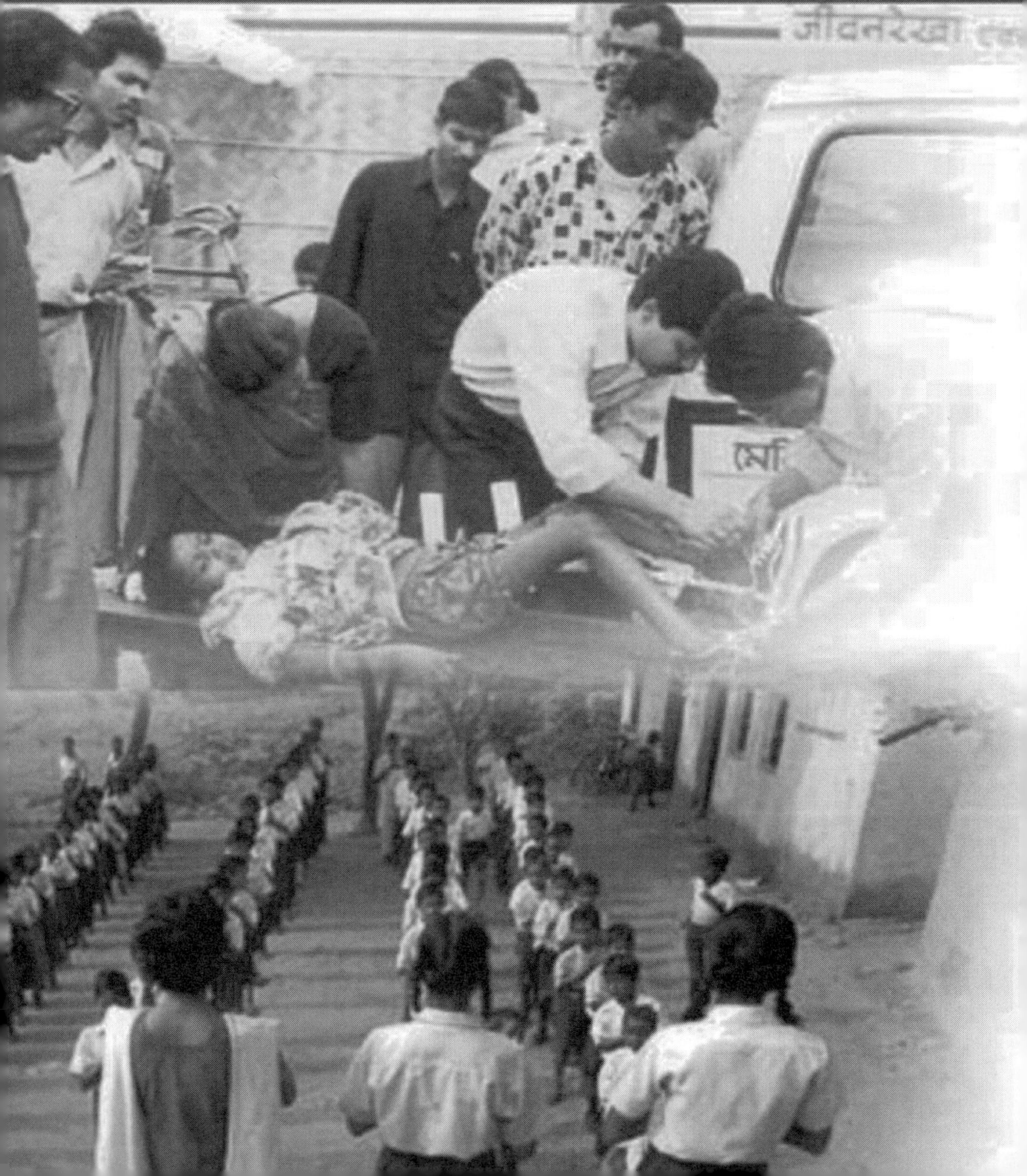
जीवनरेखा

The money that goes to charity has always been seen as a noble usage of the wealth we have created from our companies. It goes back into education, medical, alleviation of poverty or rural development.

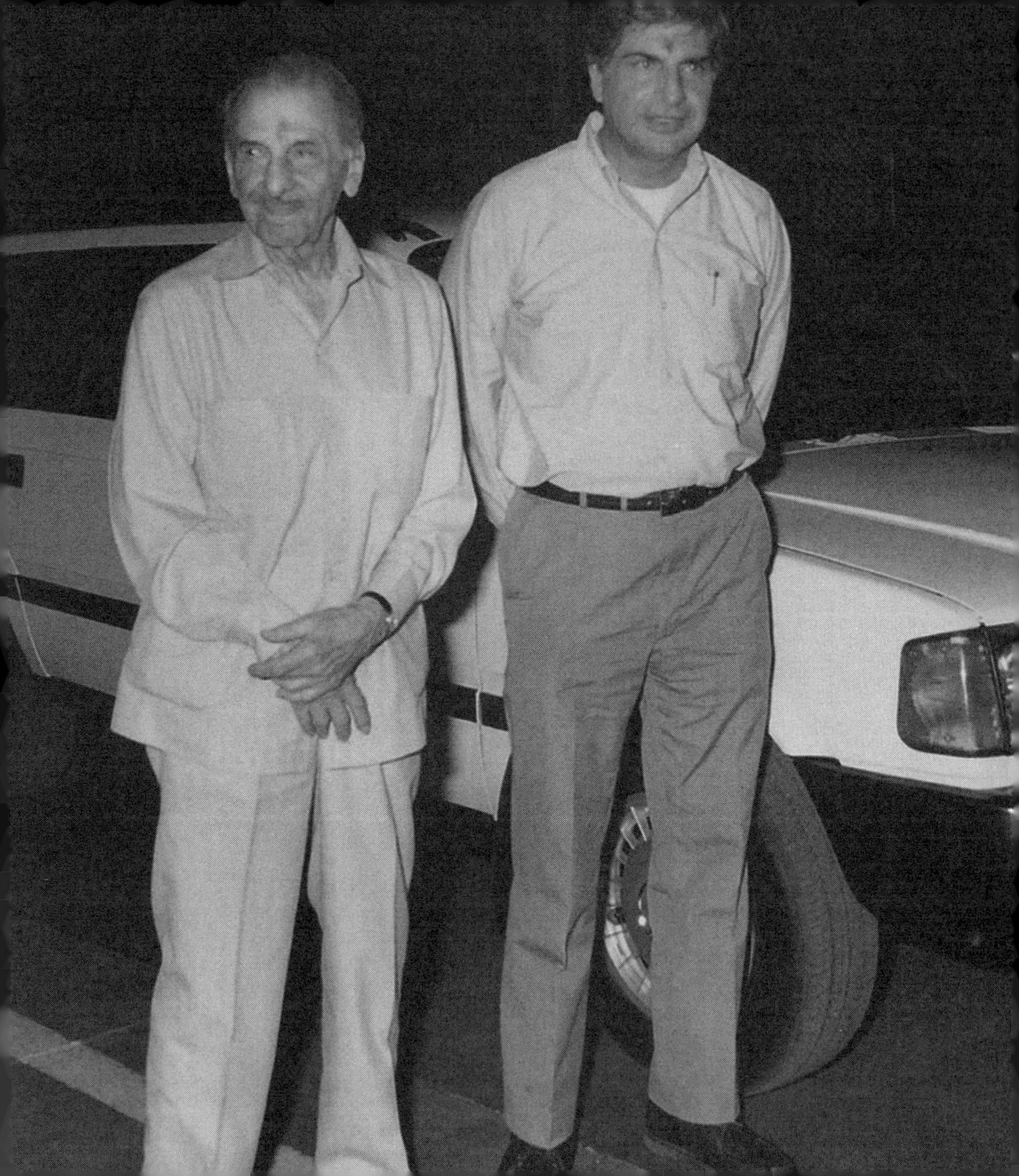

The early Rockefellers made their wealth from being in certain businesses and remained personally very wealthy. The Tatas were different, in the sense that its future generations were not so wealthy. They were involved in the business but most of the family wealth was put into trusts and most of the family did not, in fact, enjoy enormous wealth.

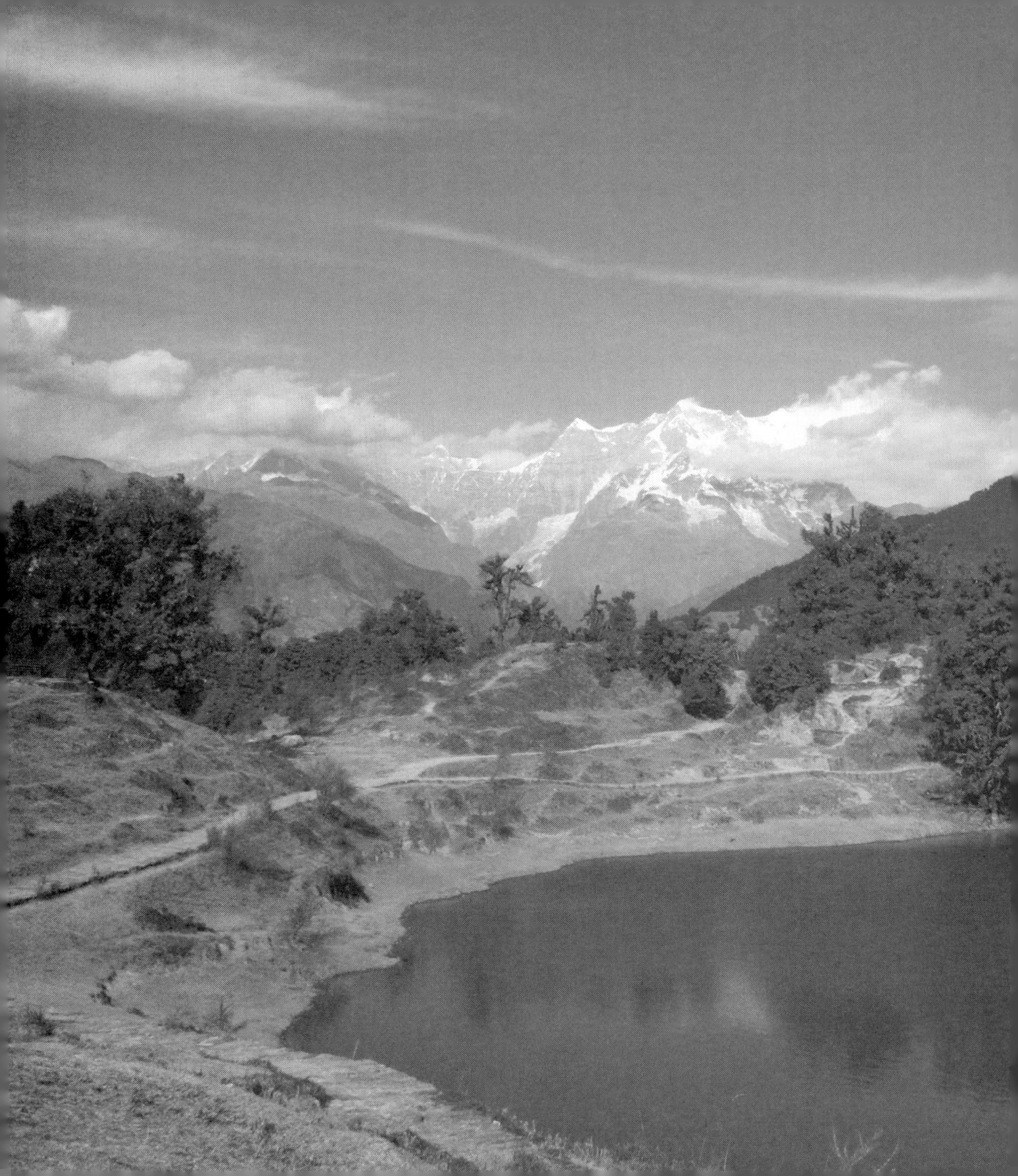

We have to be fair to all our stakeholders. Being just to every constituent of the community is crucial; it is the cornerstone of the tremendous equity that Tata products and services enjoy, and the basis of the faith and trust reposed by people in Tata.

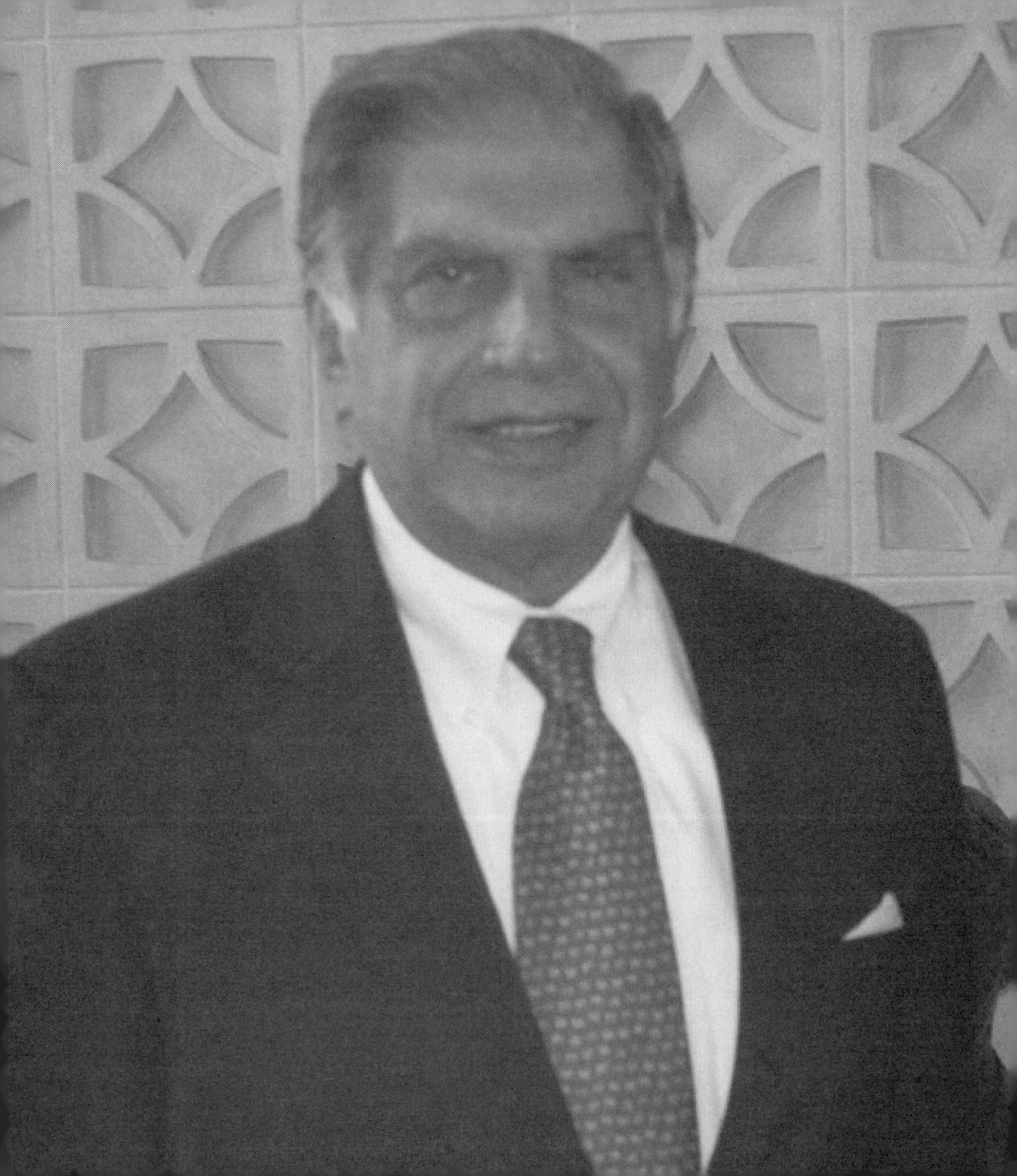

I get enormous pleasure from seeing the uplift of an underprivileged or poor person. I feel elated when I walk on the street and see someone who pushes a handcart talking on a cellphone.

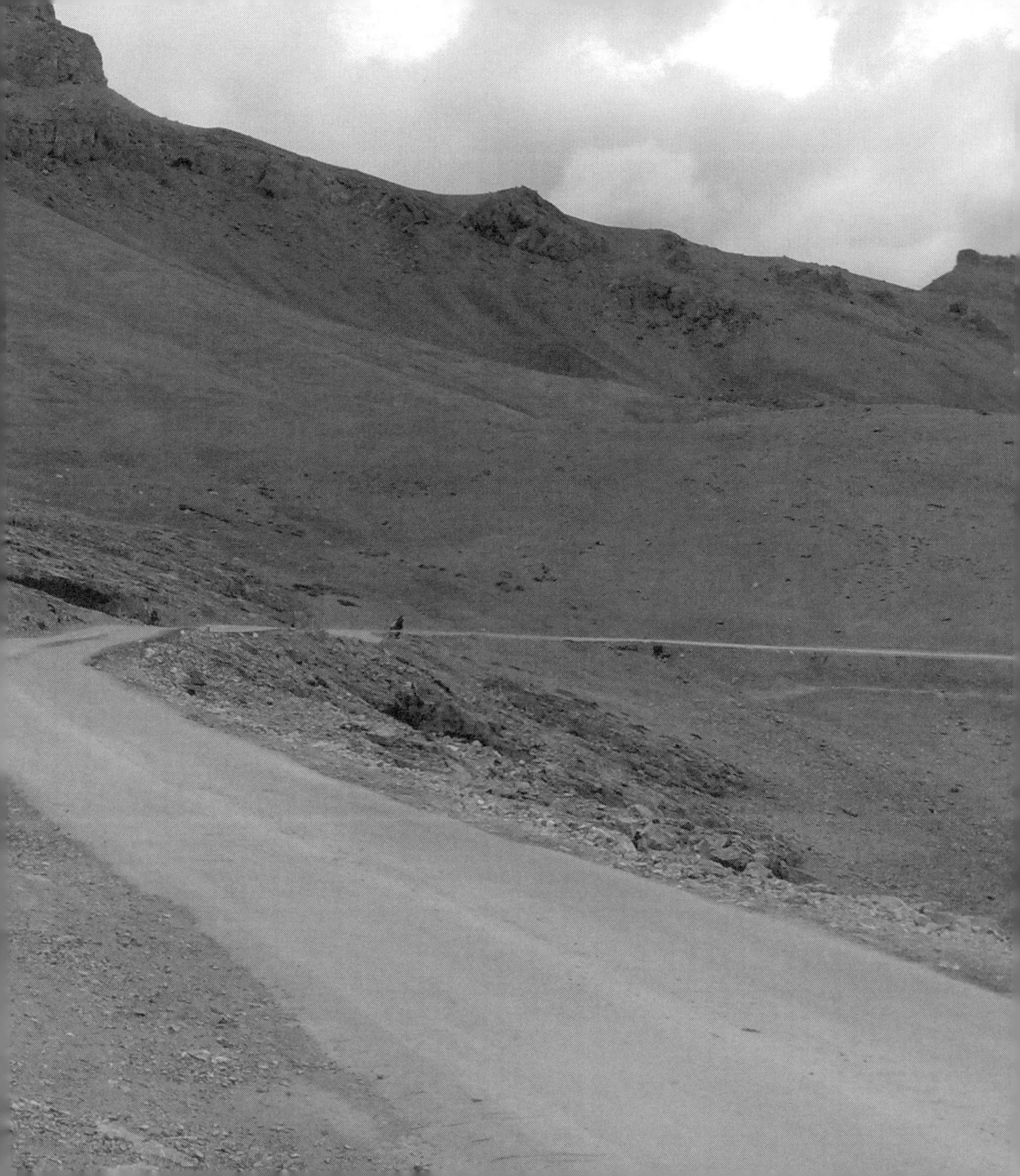

Philanthropic institutions in India still believe they are charitable and therefore must operate on shoestring budgets, that creating an organisation is almost a luxury. This thinking needs to change; they have to recognise that a non-profit has as much responsibility for being professionally run as a corporate body.

INDIA STORY

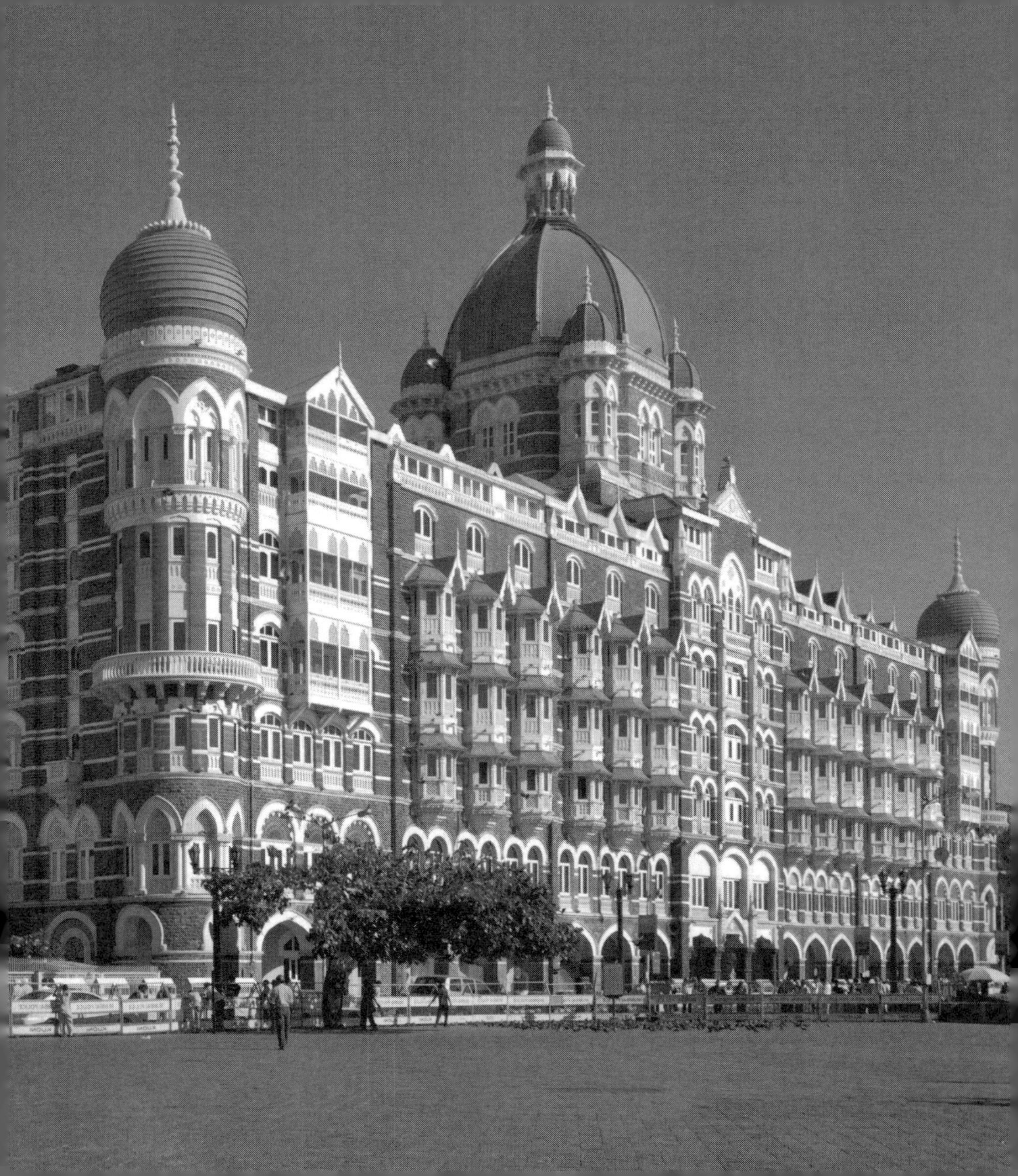

I think the Tata group's greatest contribution to the growth of the Indian economy and Indian industry probably happened in the pre-independence era. The group's investments in industries such as steel, textiles, power and hotels were certainly driven by an entrepreneurial spirit, but they were driven even more by a desire to make India self-sufficient and independent of its colonial masters.

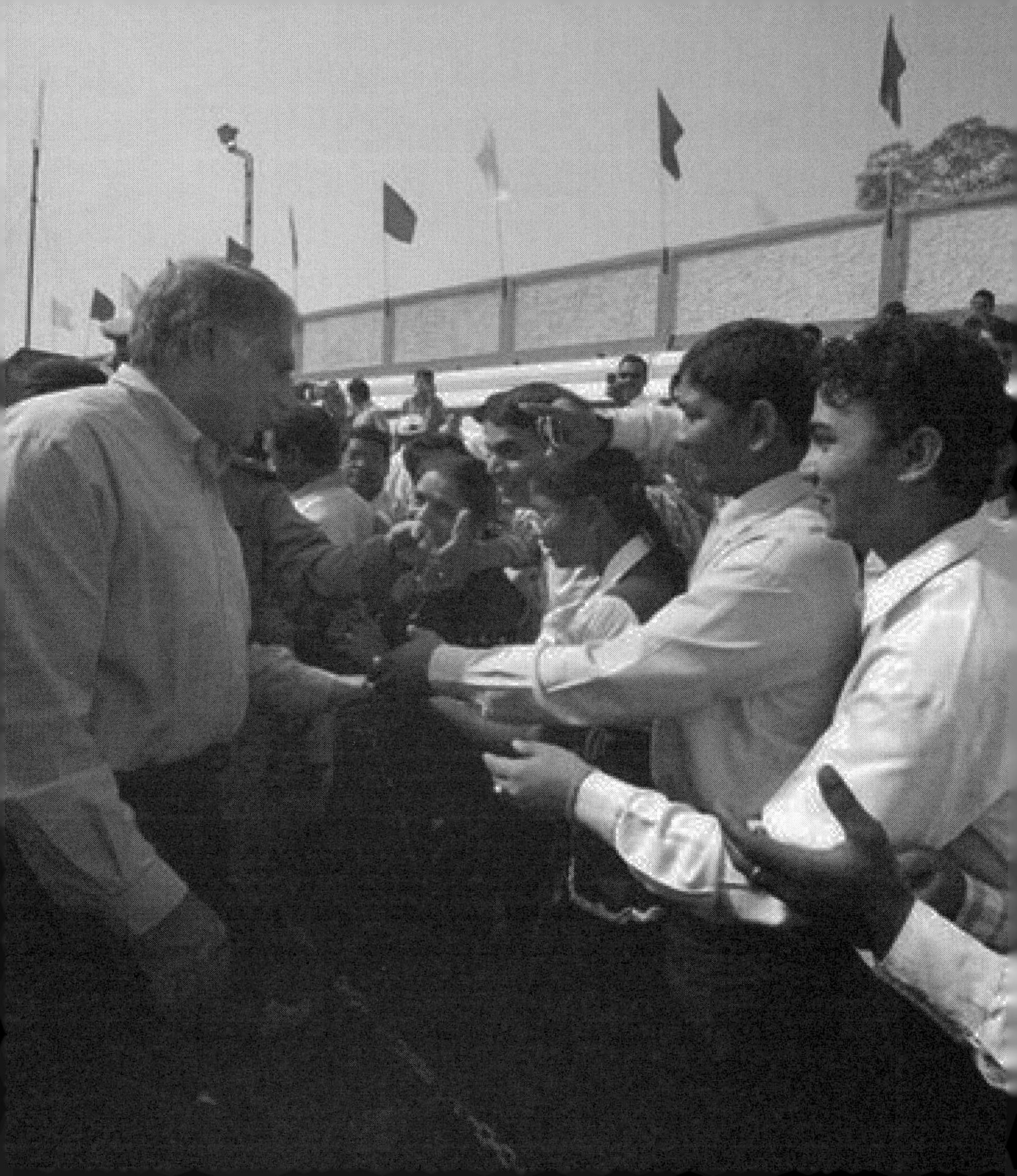

I am proud of my country. But we need to unite to create a unified India, free of communalism and caste. We need to build India into a land of equal opportunity for all.

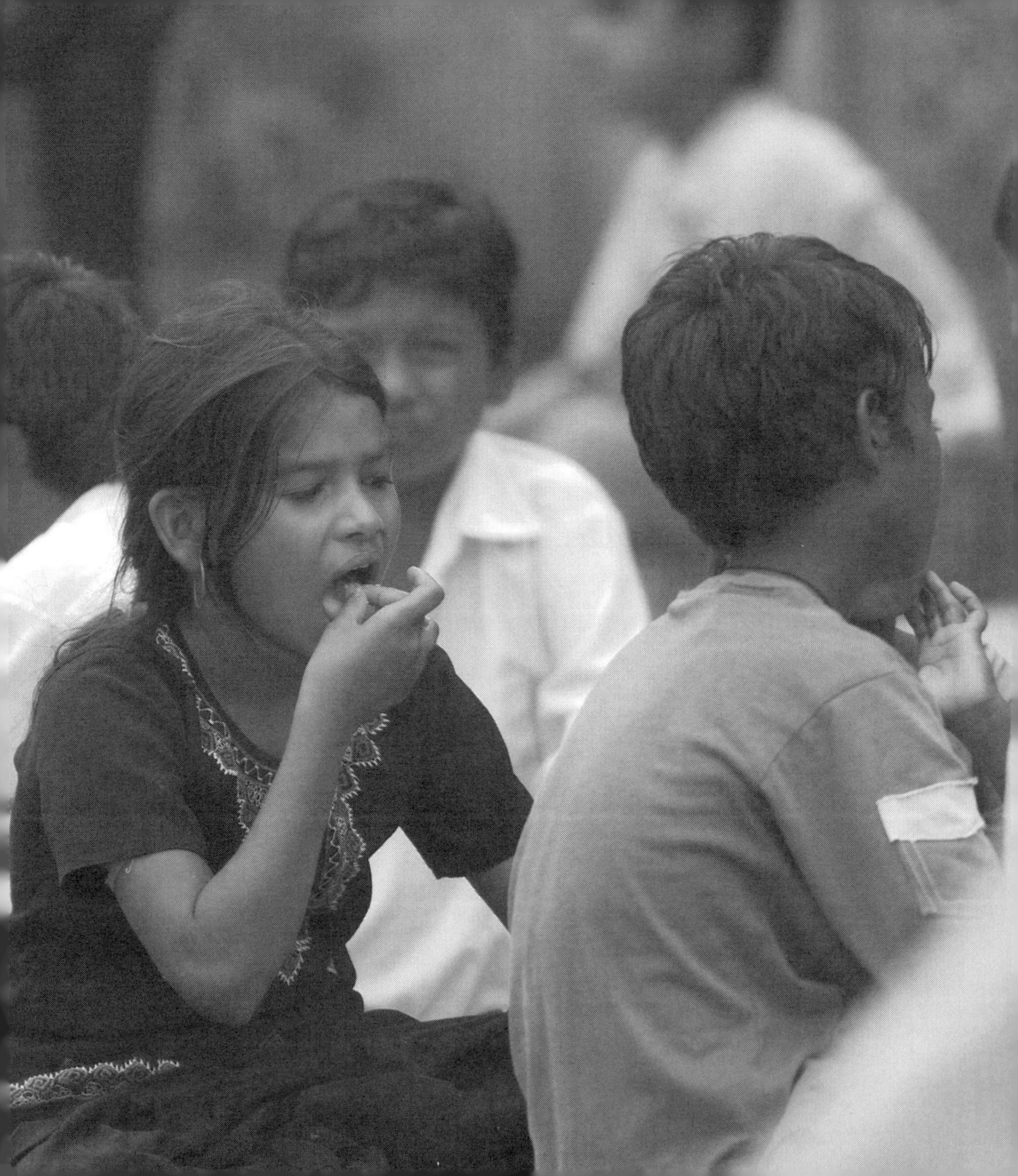

I feel very sensitive and concerned about people who have been traditionally deprived but the word 'caste' is not in my vocabulary at all.

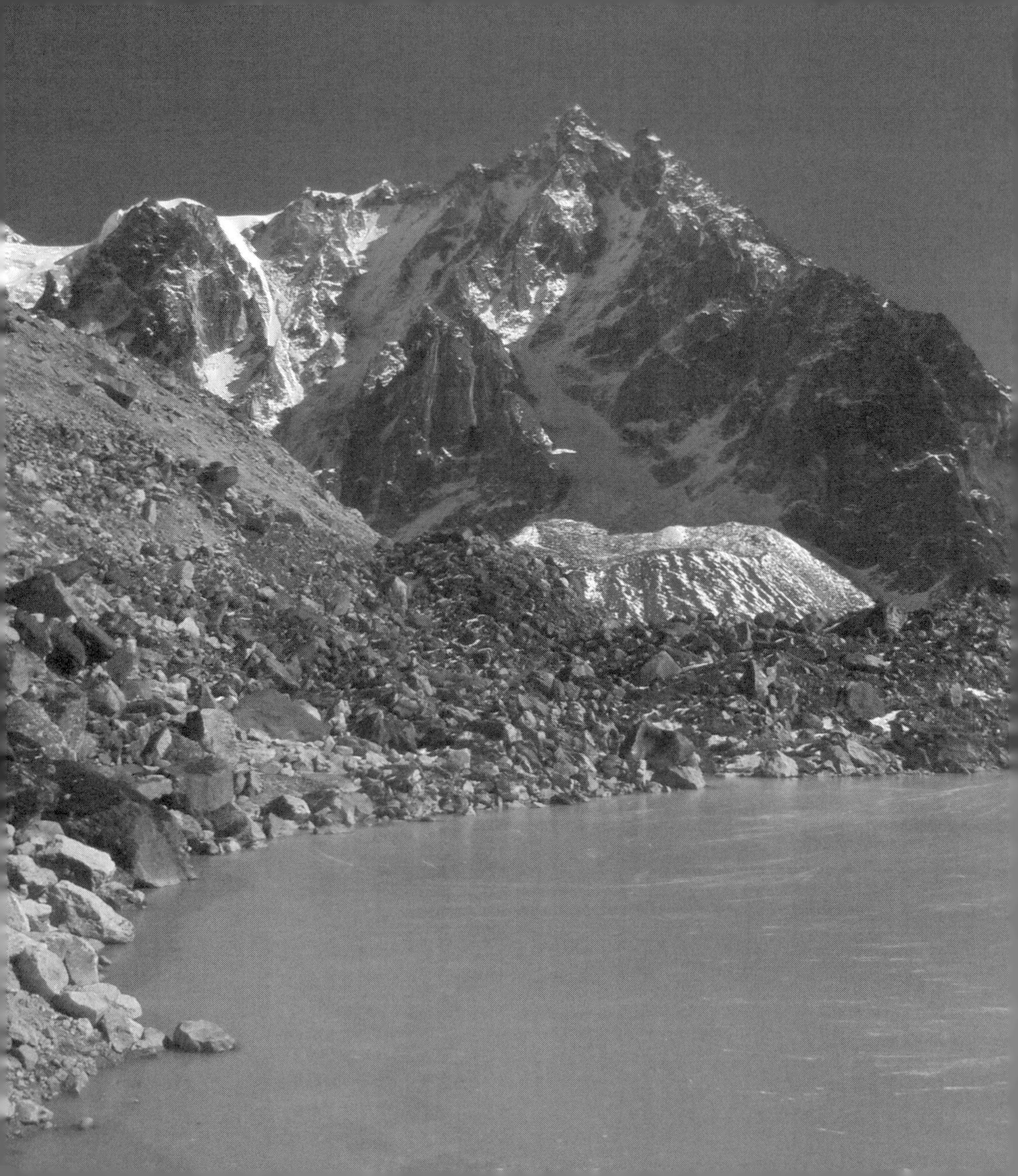

We can be a truly great nation if we set our sights high and deliver to the people the fruits of continued growth, prosperity and equal opportunity.

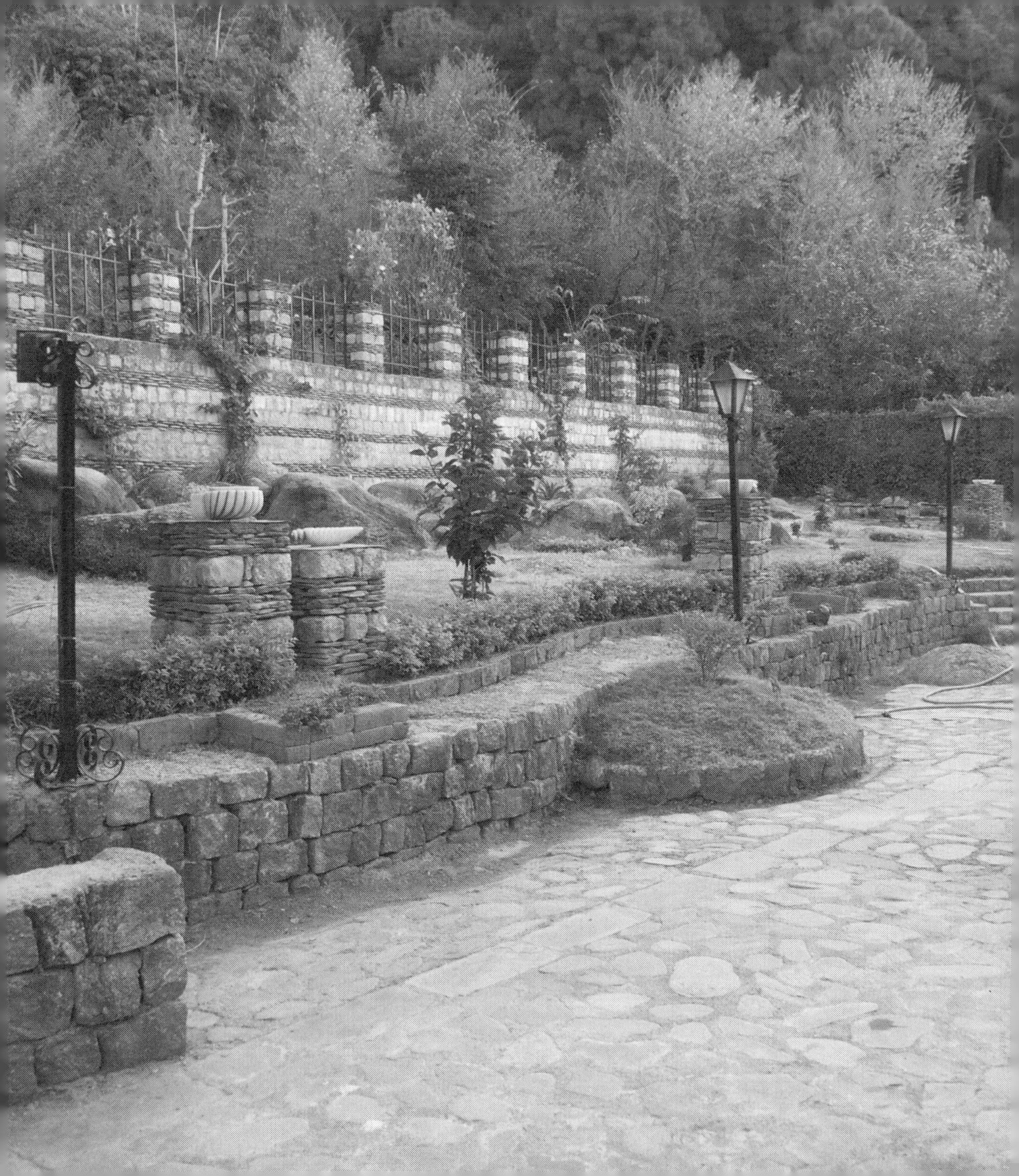

In rural India, too, the quality of life has without any doubt improved. We still have great disparities and it would be false to say that everything is fine. But it would also be wrong to say that India hasn't moved; it has moved a great distance.

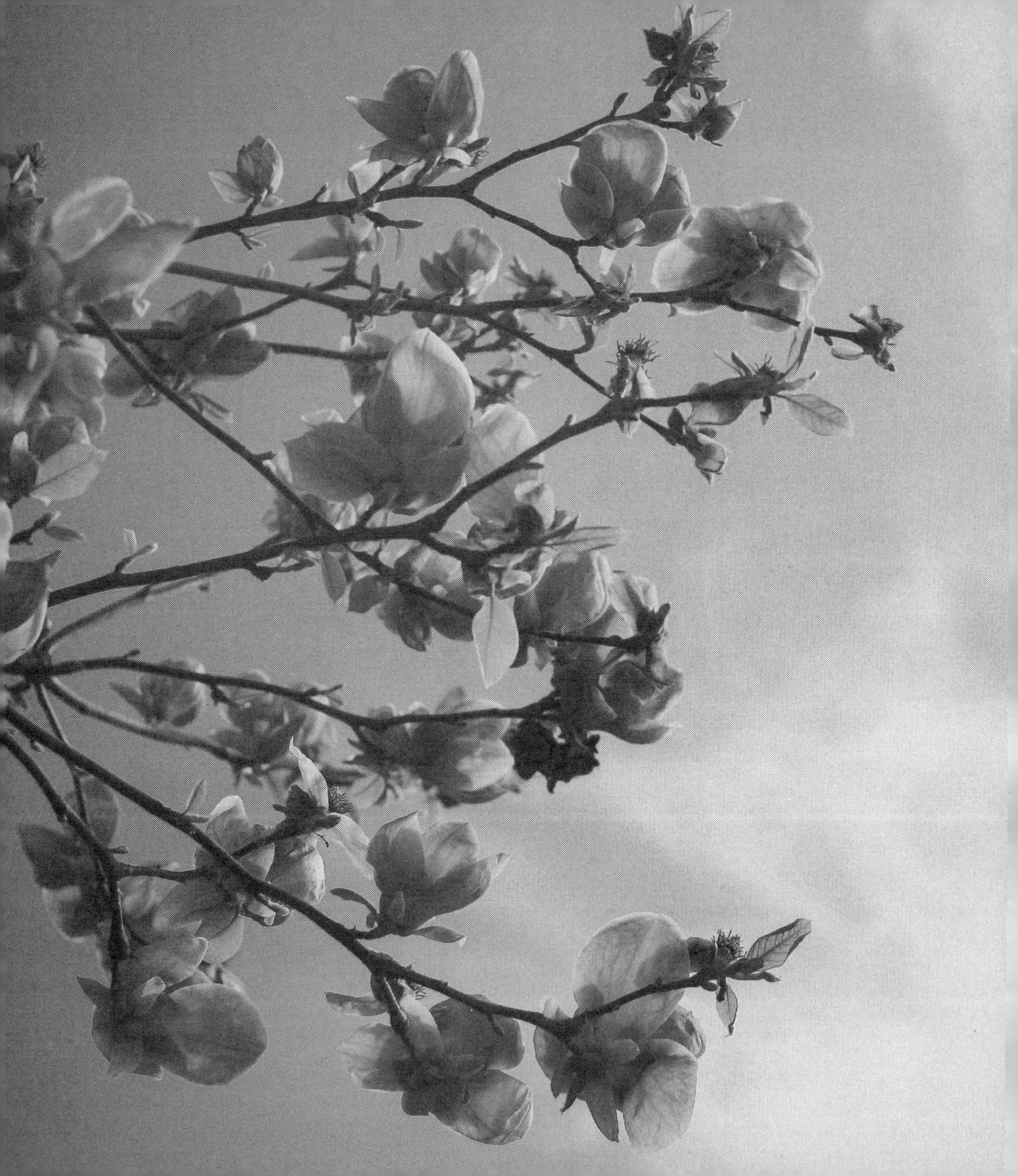

India is now universally recognised as a nation on the move and takes its place amongst the successful economies in the region. The future potential is enormous and the country's destiny is in our hands.

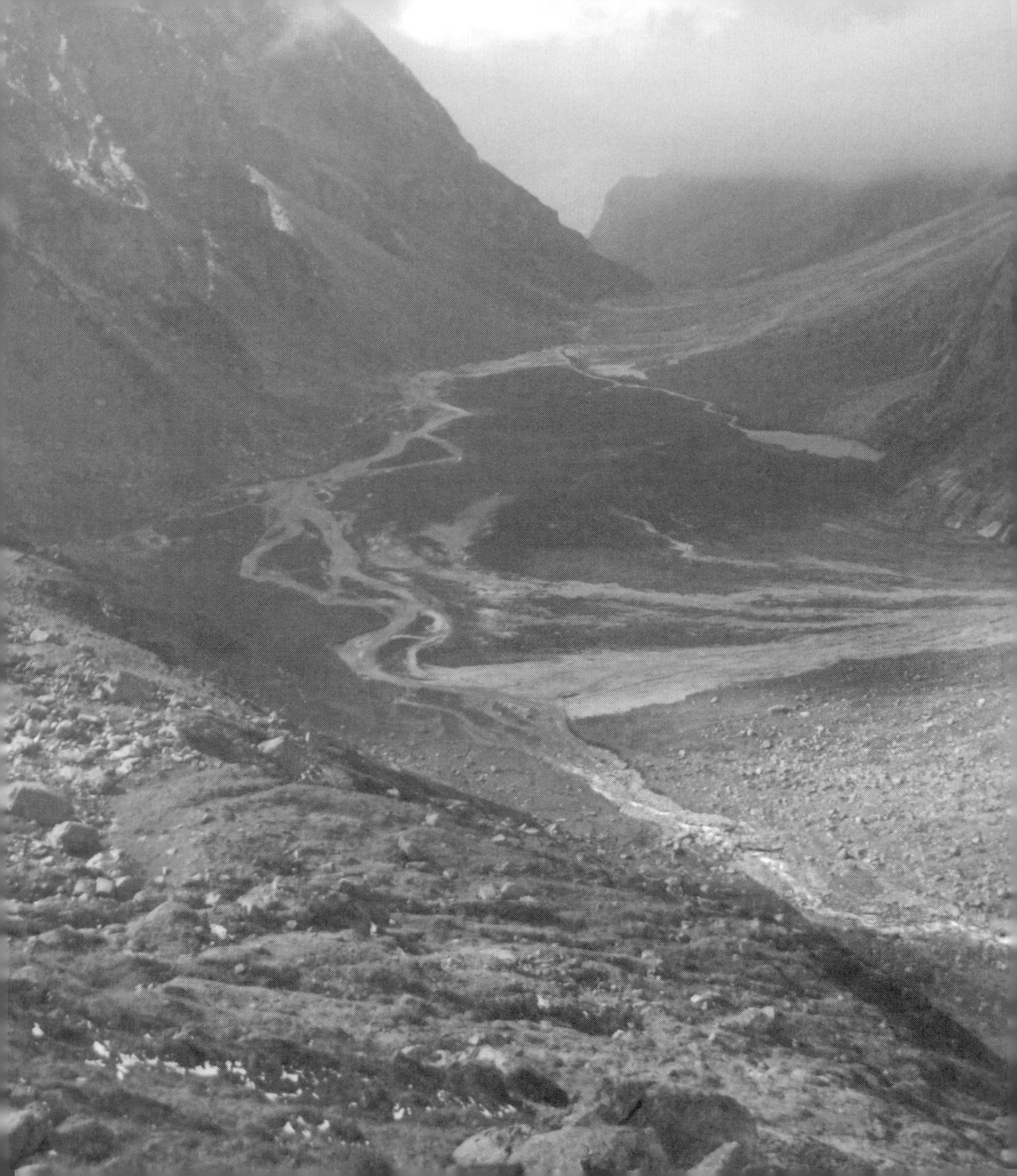

In a developing country such as India, we should perhaps be more active in shedding some of the old baggage and embracing new opportunities.

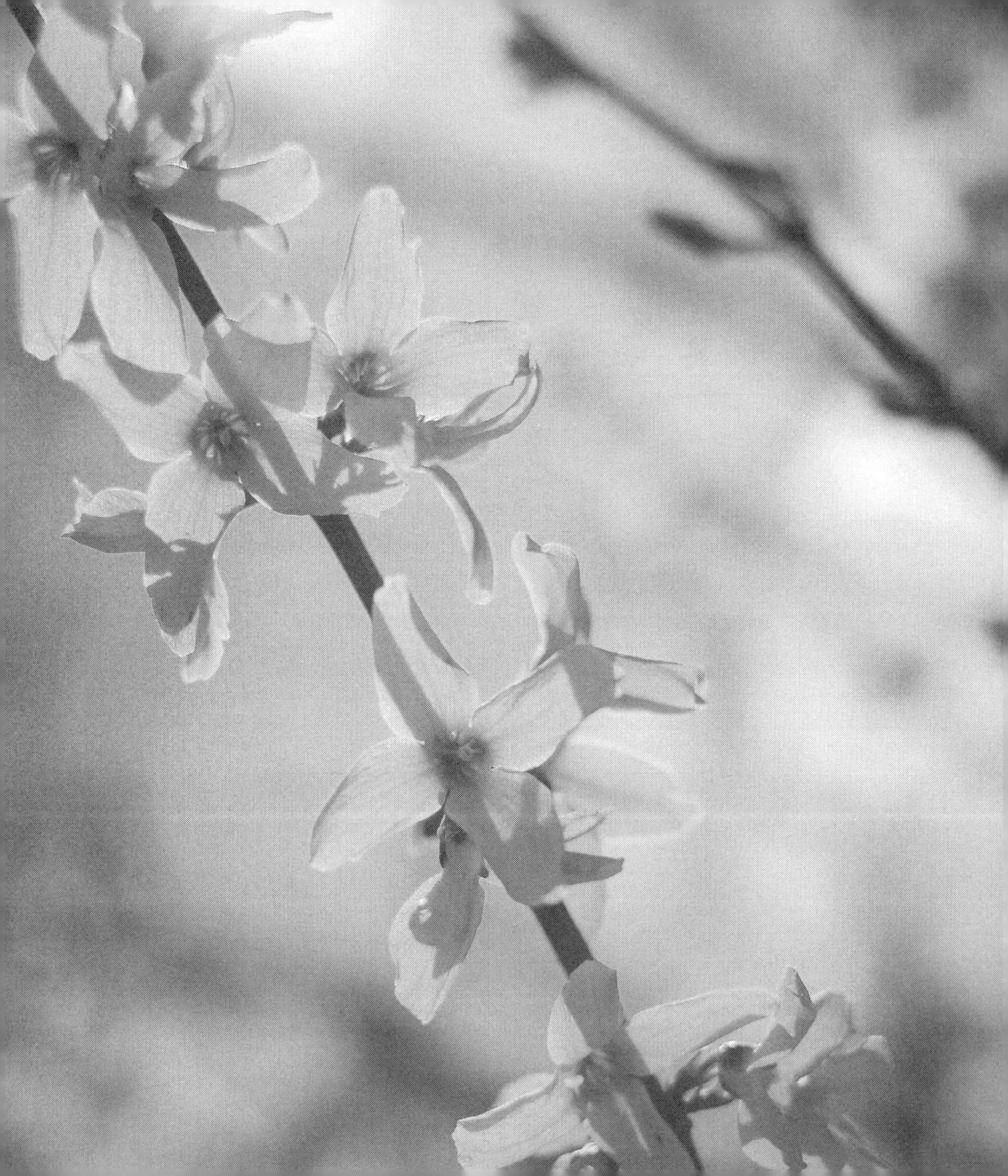

We never really plan big. We are not in step with what is happening around us. When you go to other countries, you see it visibly that we are just back in time. And yet we have so much to offer.

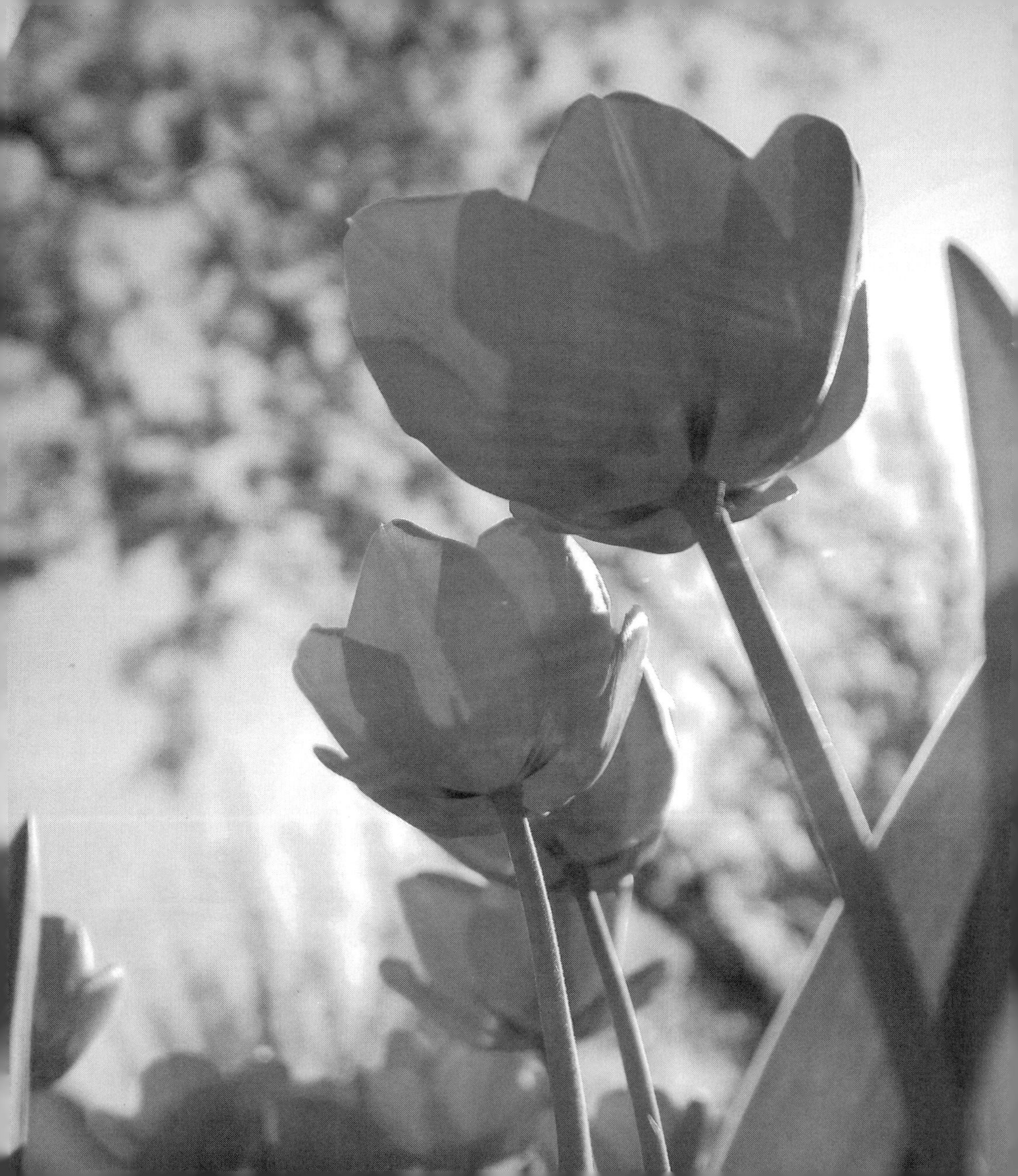

I feel India is a country that really has an enormous amount of potential, has the human capital to succeed. But if you sit down and ask, 'Will it succeed,' then you begin to see imbalances.

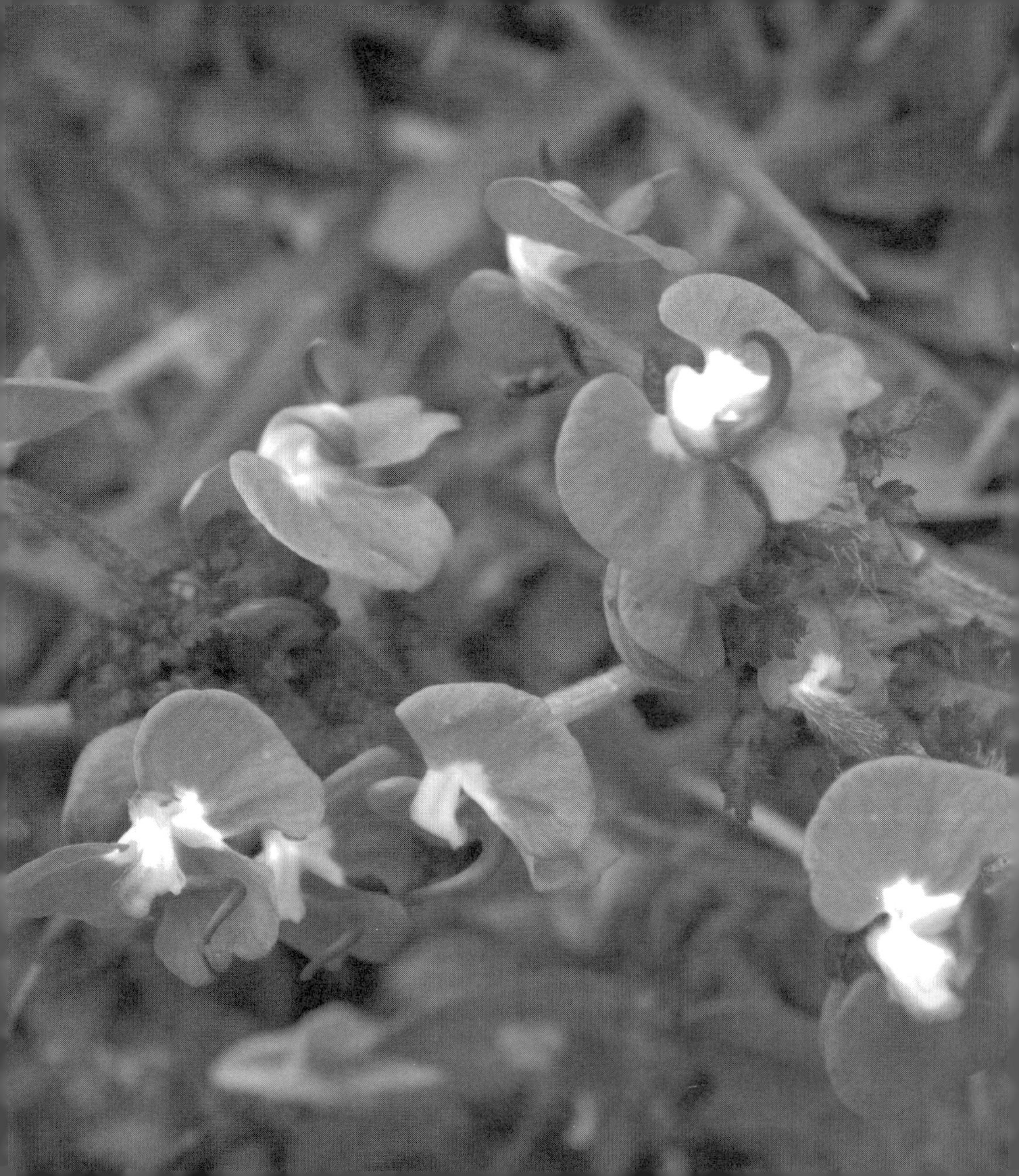

The vision I have for India in the next decade is of a nation with vastly improved connectivity in communications providing education, personal interaction, e-commerce, and telephony contact for the overwhelming mass of its people. I see our country being connected through major highway networks, thus shrinking the time required to move goods to the marketplace. I see our consumers exercising an unprecedented degree of choice, with the Indian marketplace becoming a vibrantly competitive arena, fully integrated with the world. Equally, I foresee that the ambitions of the Indian entrepreneur will not be confined to domestic boundaries and our immensely valuable human capital will leave its mark in the global marketplace.

(2008)

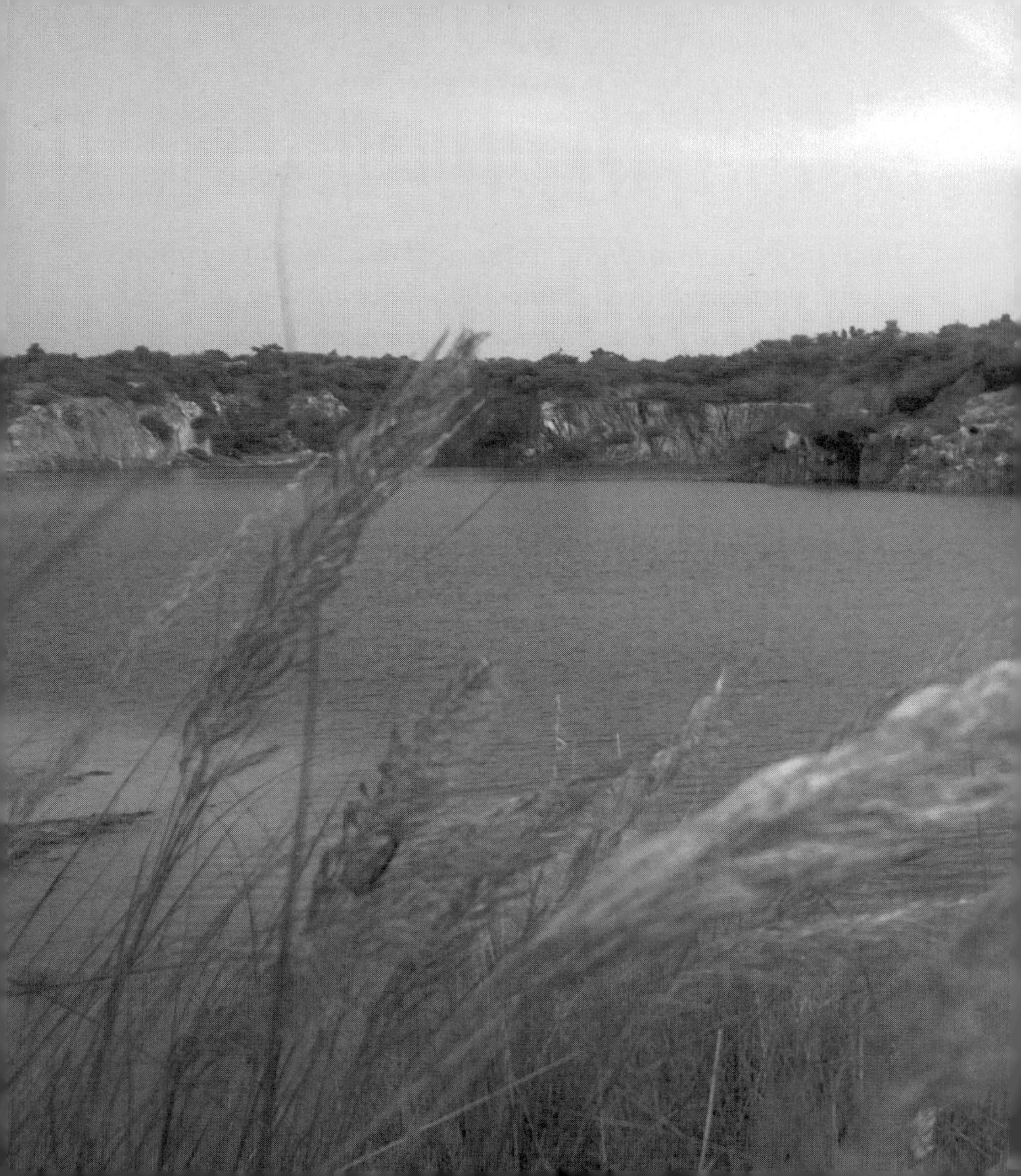

The time has come to move from small increments to bold, large initiatives. The time has come to stretch the envelope and set goals which were earlier not seen to be achievable. The time has come for performance to be measured and for allocated funds of the government to reach the people for whom they are intended.

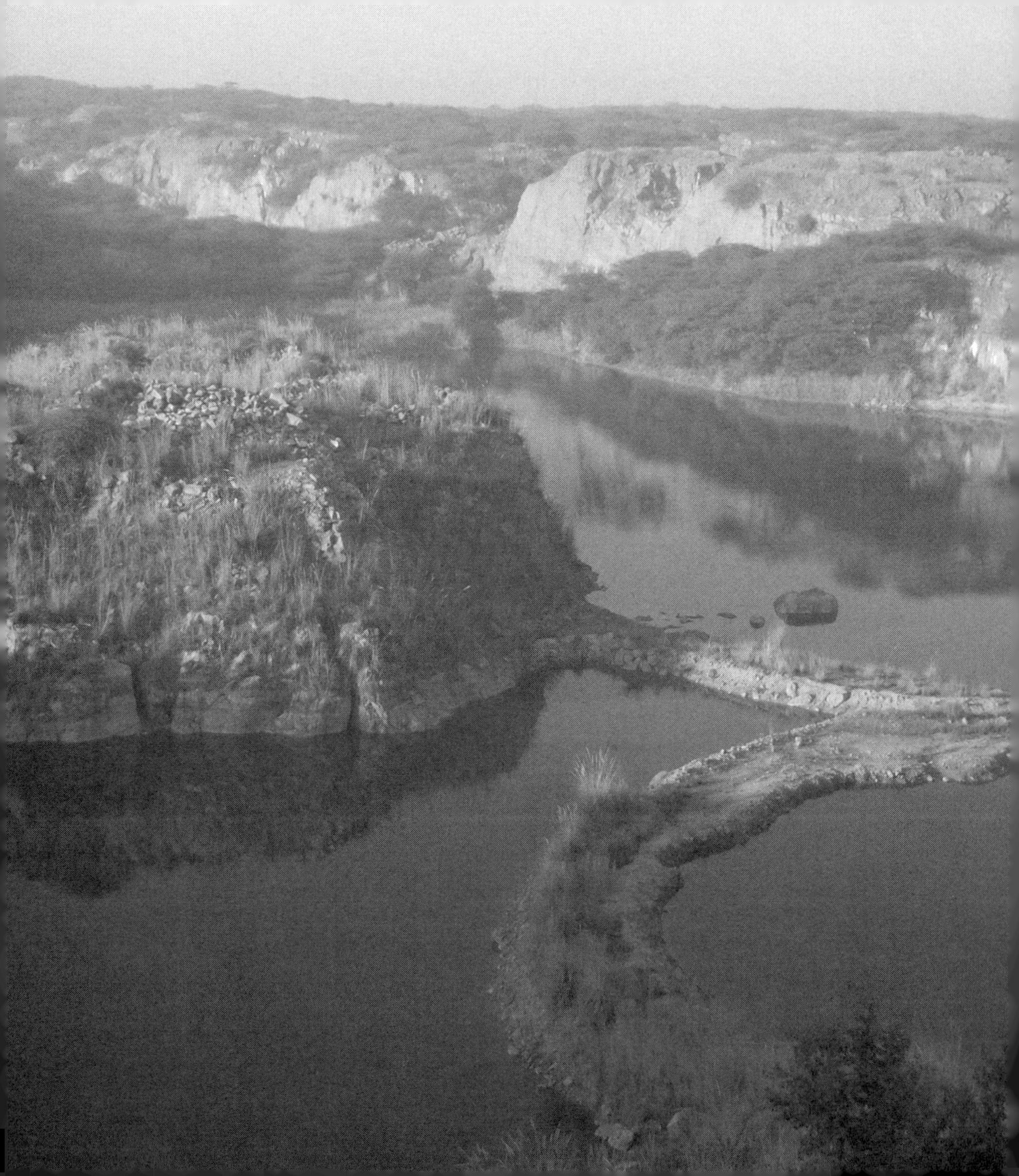

We have been thinking small. Countries like China have grown so much by thinking big. I would urge that we all think big, think of doing things not in small increments, not in small deltas, but seemingly impossible things. Nothing is impossible if you really set out to accomplish things and if you act boldly. Because it is this thinking big and acting boldly that will move India up in a manner different from what obtains today.

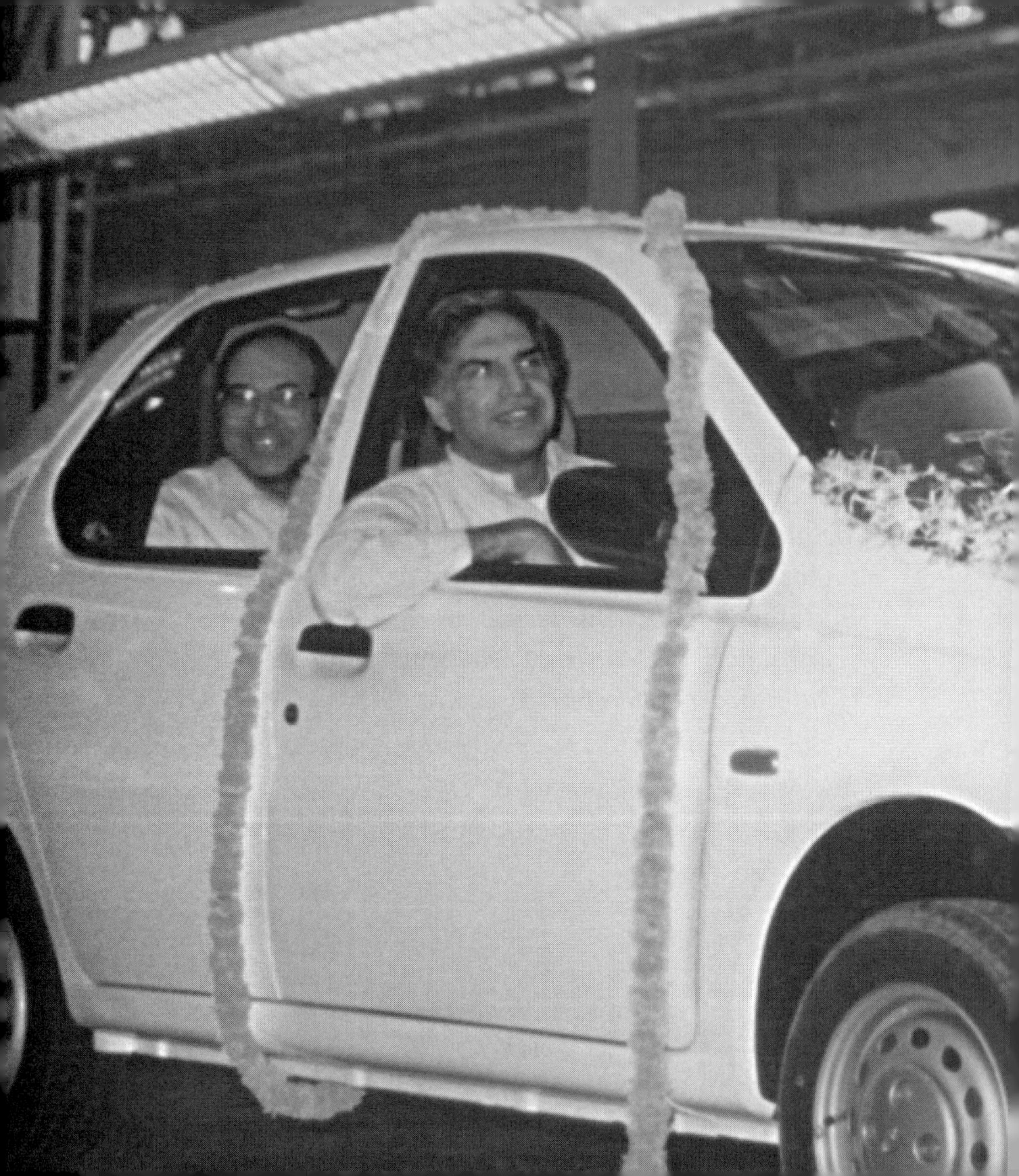

My only regret is that I am not 20 years younger, because I think India is going through a very exciting period in its history.

LIFE

AND ITS

CHALLENGES

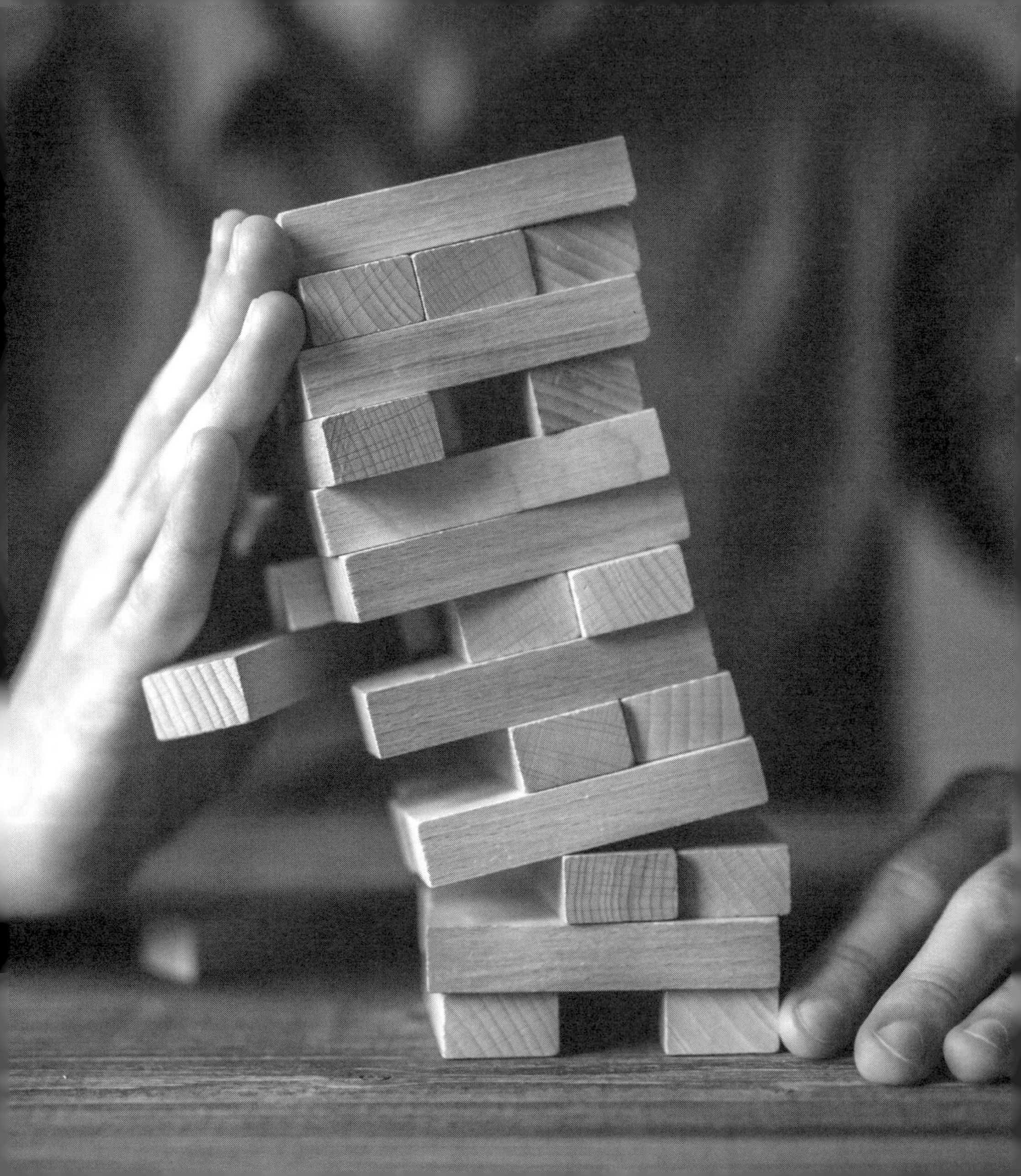

*The biggest risk is not taking any risk.
In a world that is changing quickly,
the only strategy that is guaranteed to fail
is not taking risks.*

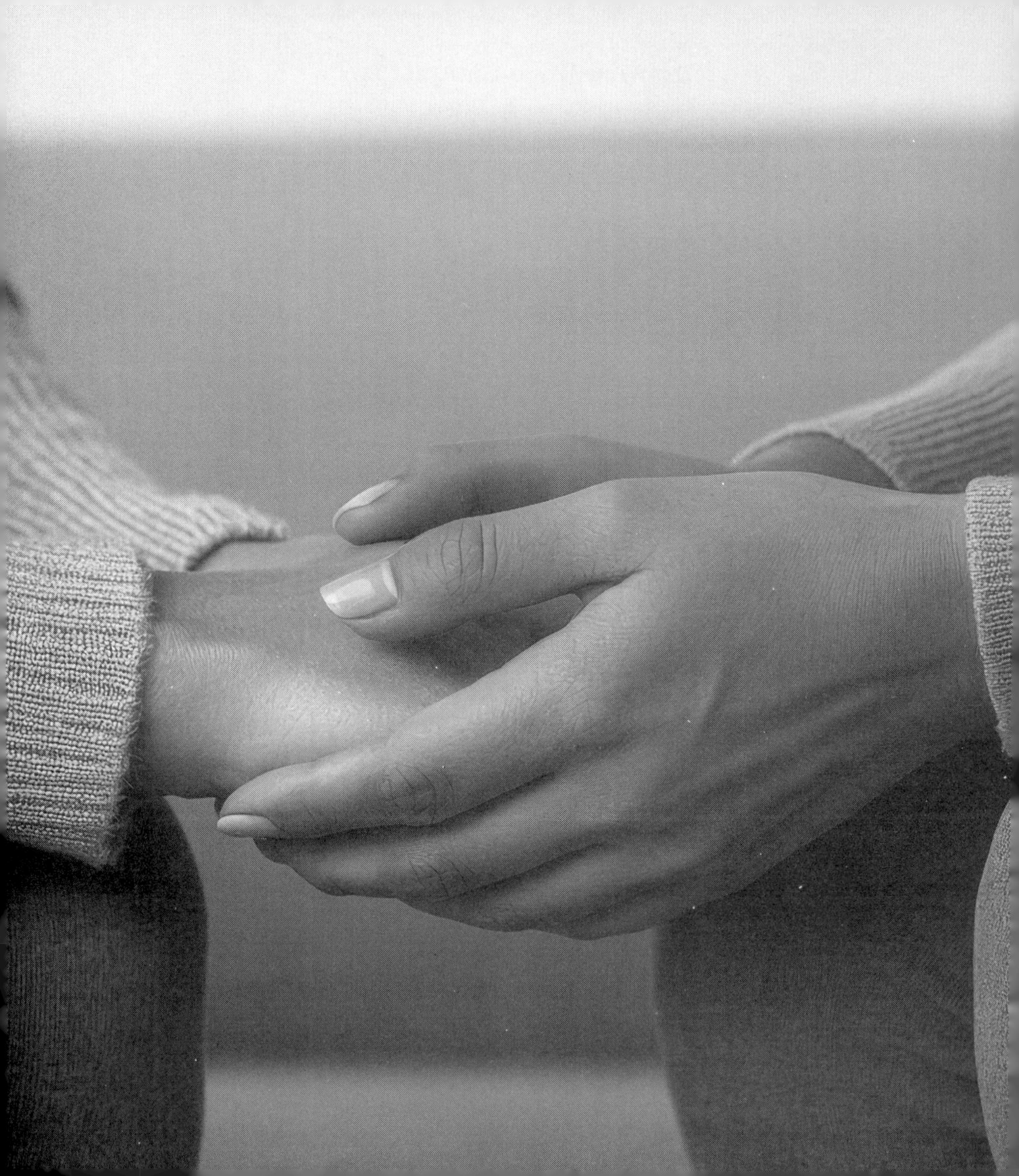

Never underestimate the power of kindness, empathy, and compassion in your interactions with others.

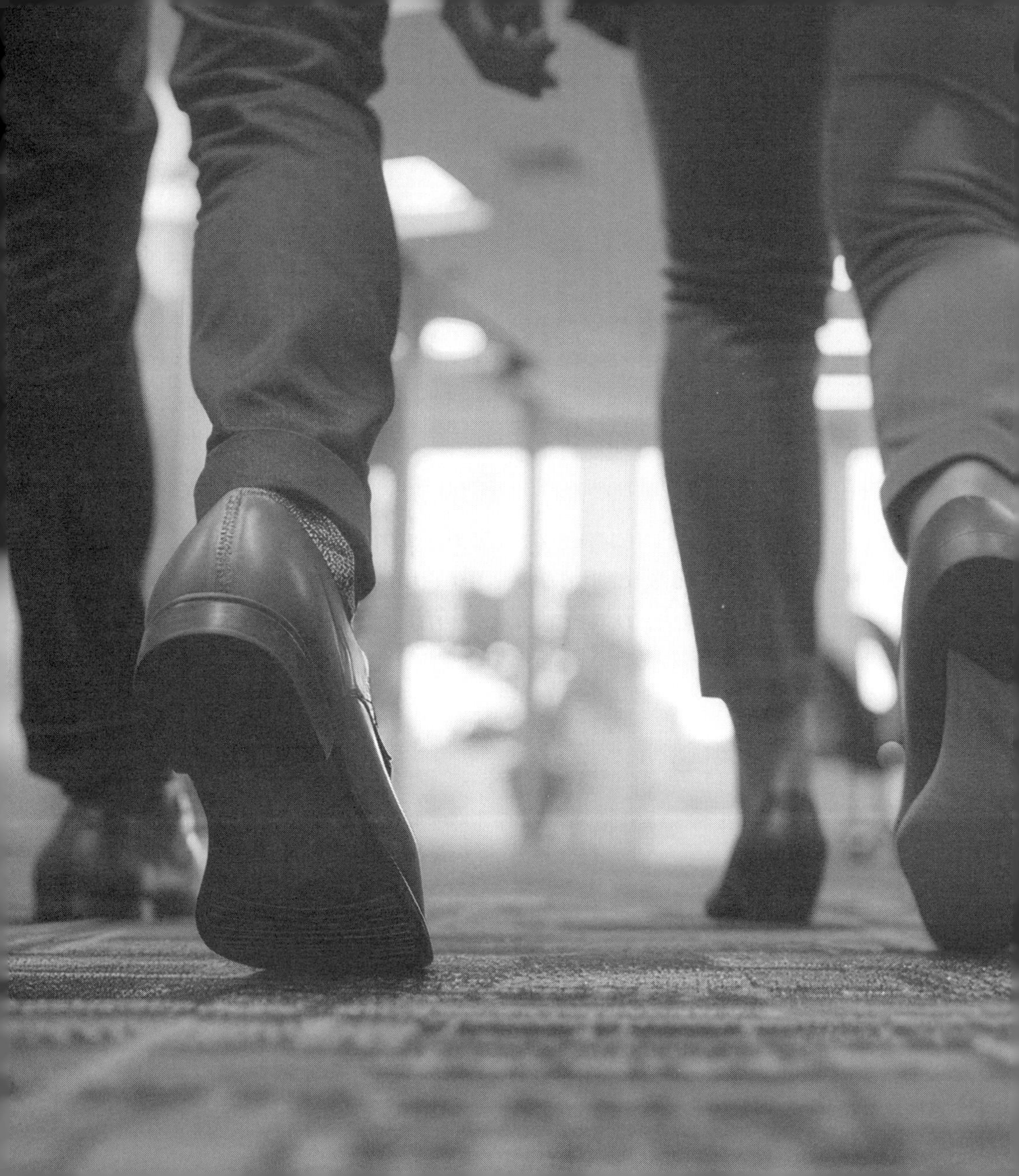

If you want to walk fast, walk alone.
But if you want to walk far, walk together.

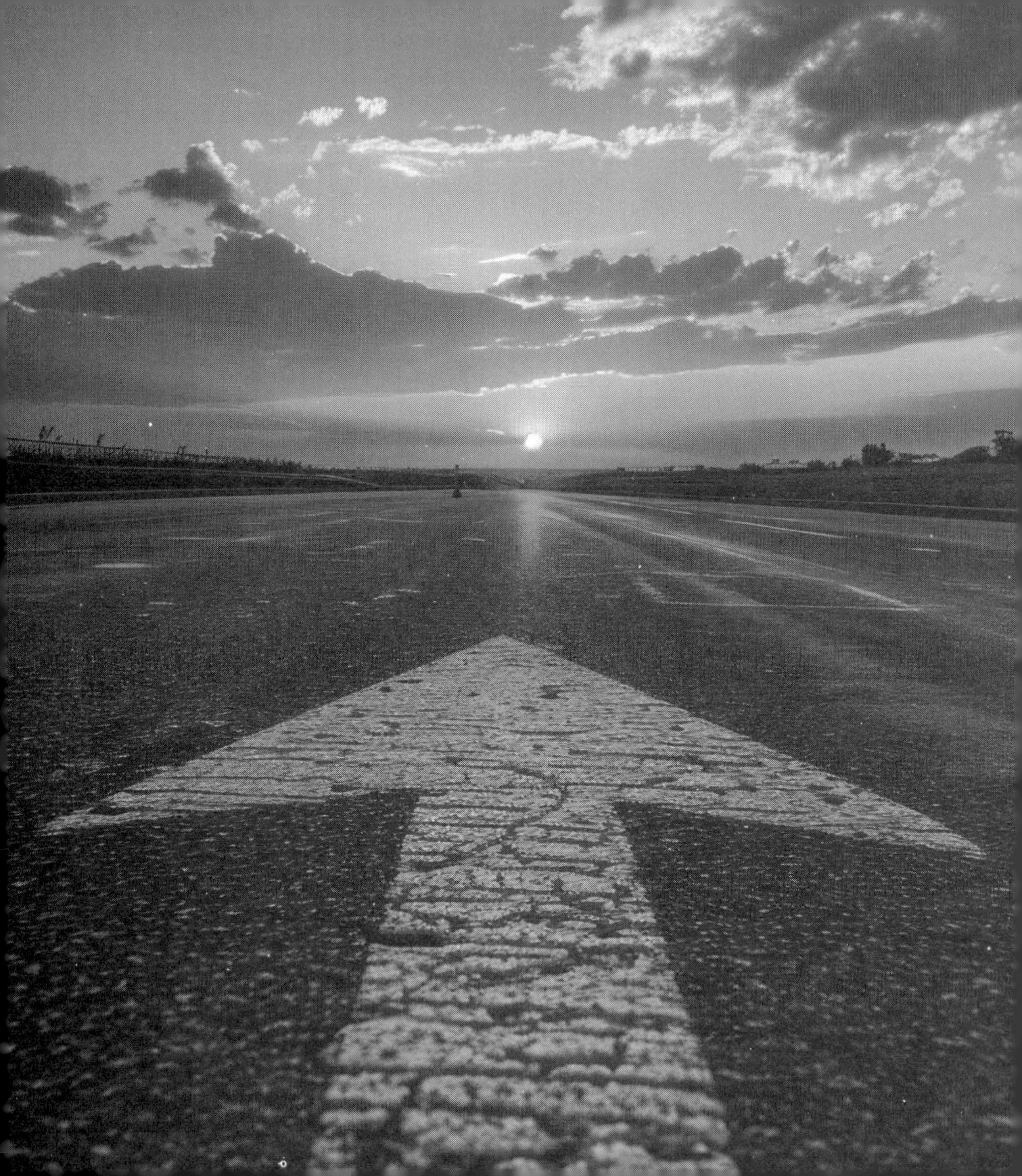

Don't wait for opportunities to come to you,
create your own opportunities.

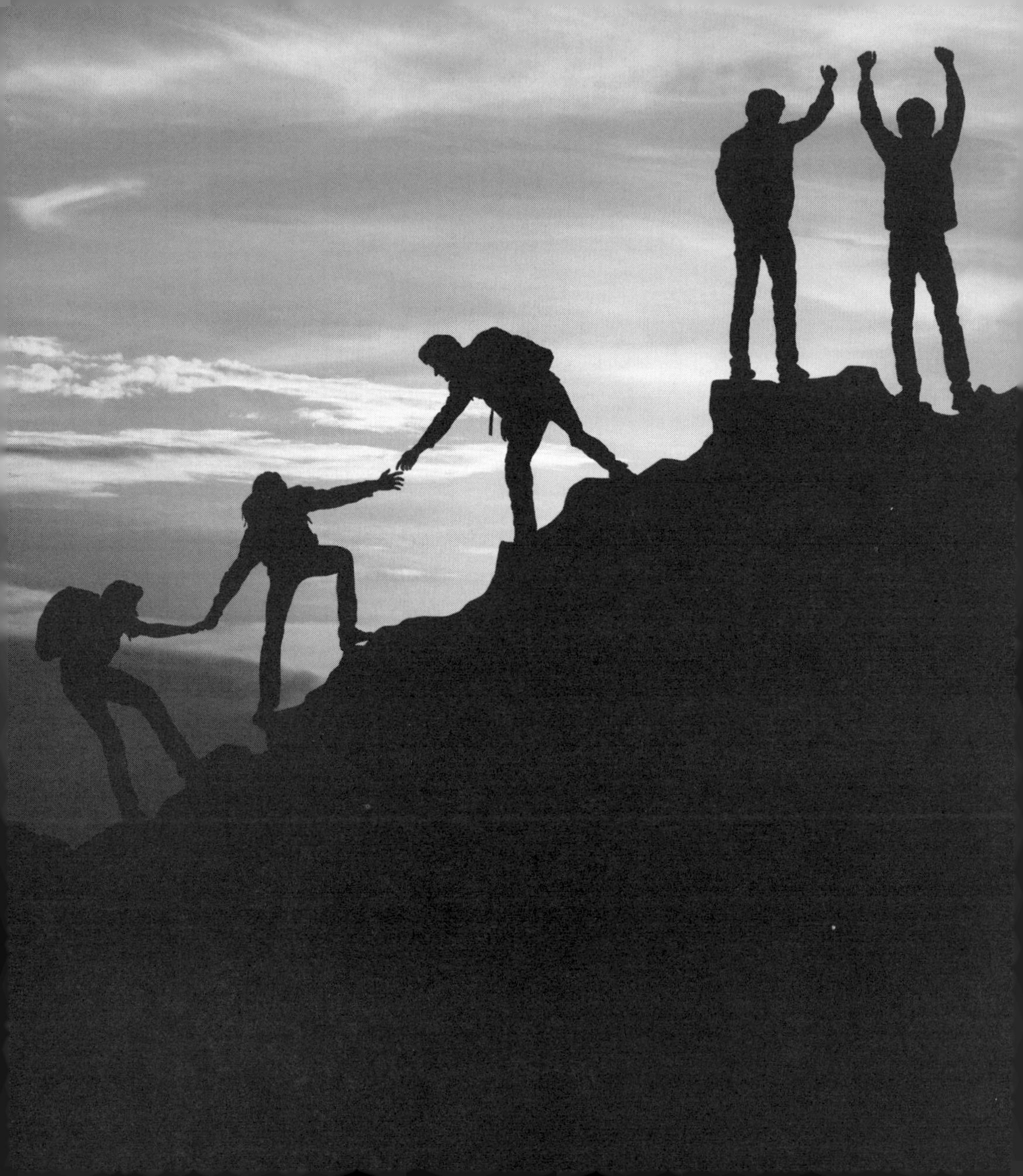

Be persistent and resilient in the face of challenges, for they are the building blocks of success.

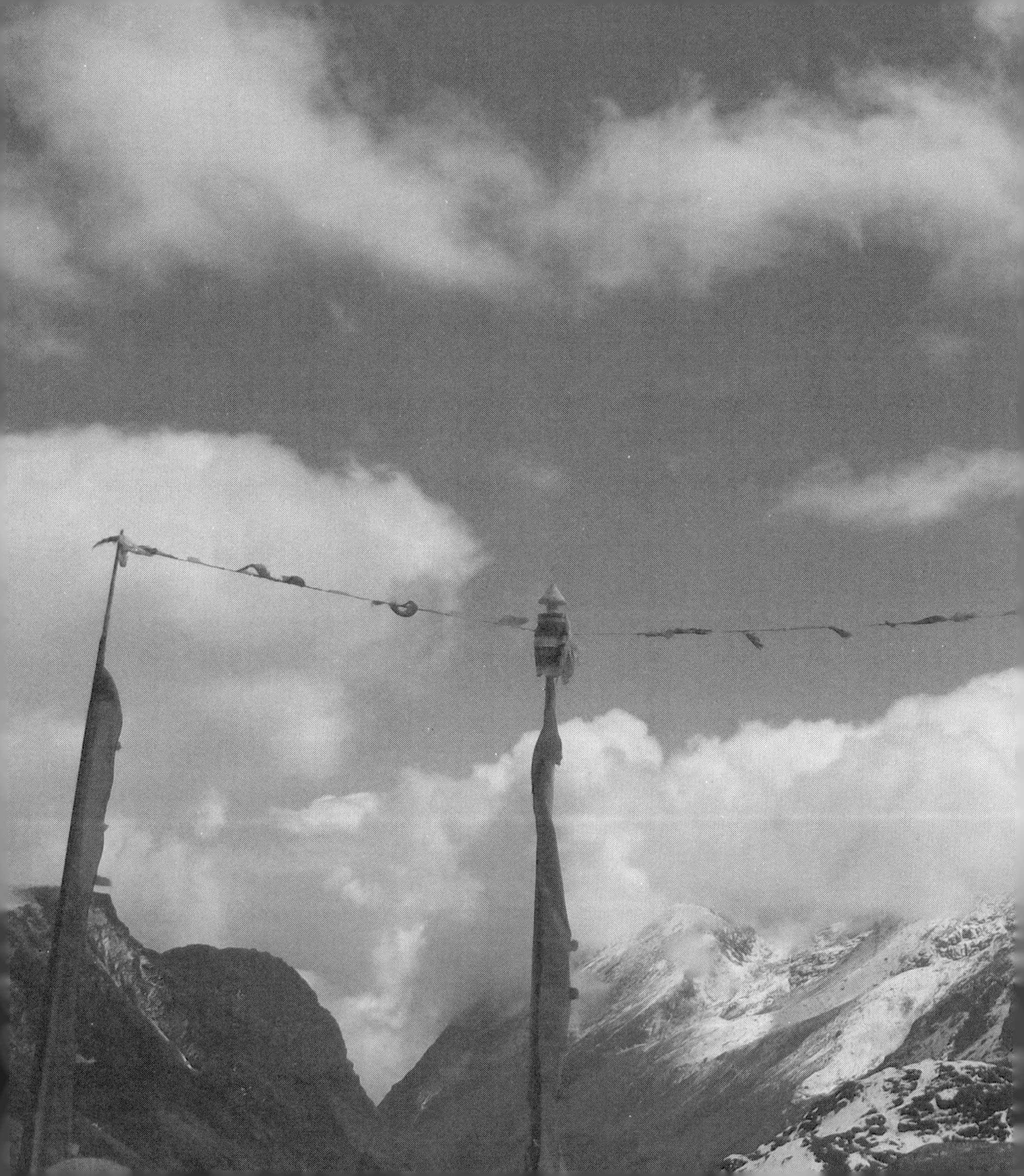

You will probably find the resistance (to change) more from those who haven't been doing well.

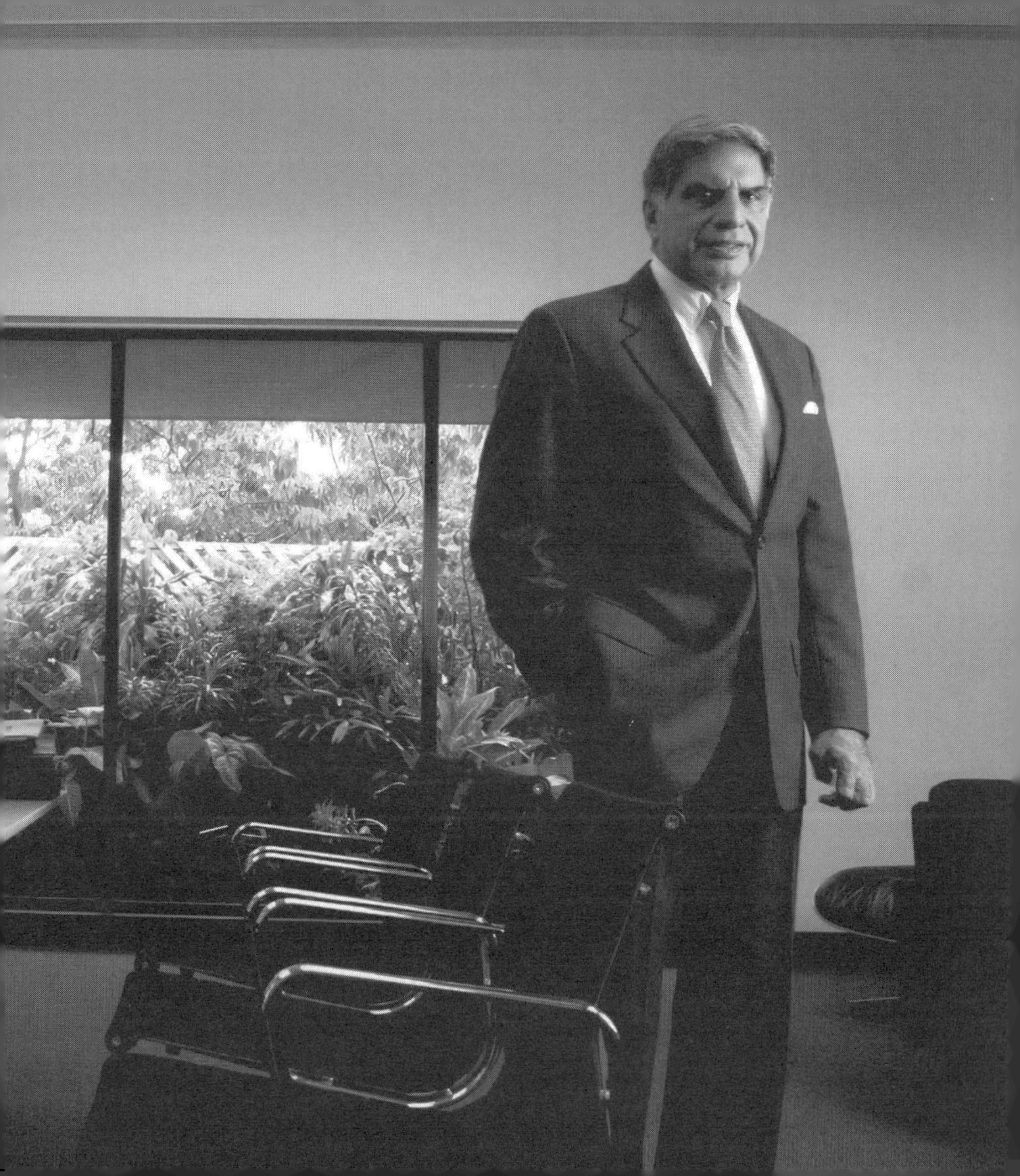

Take the stones people throw at you.
And use them to build monuments.

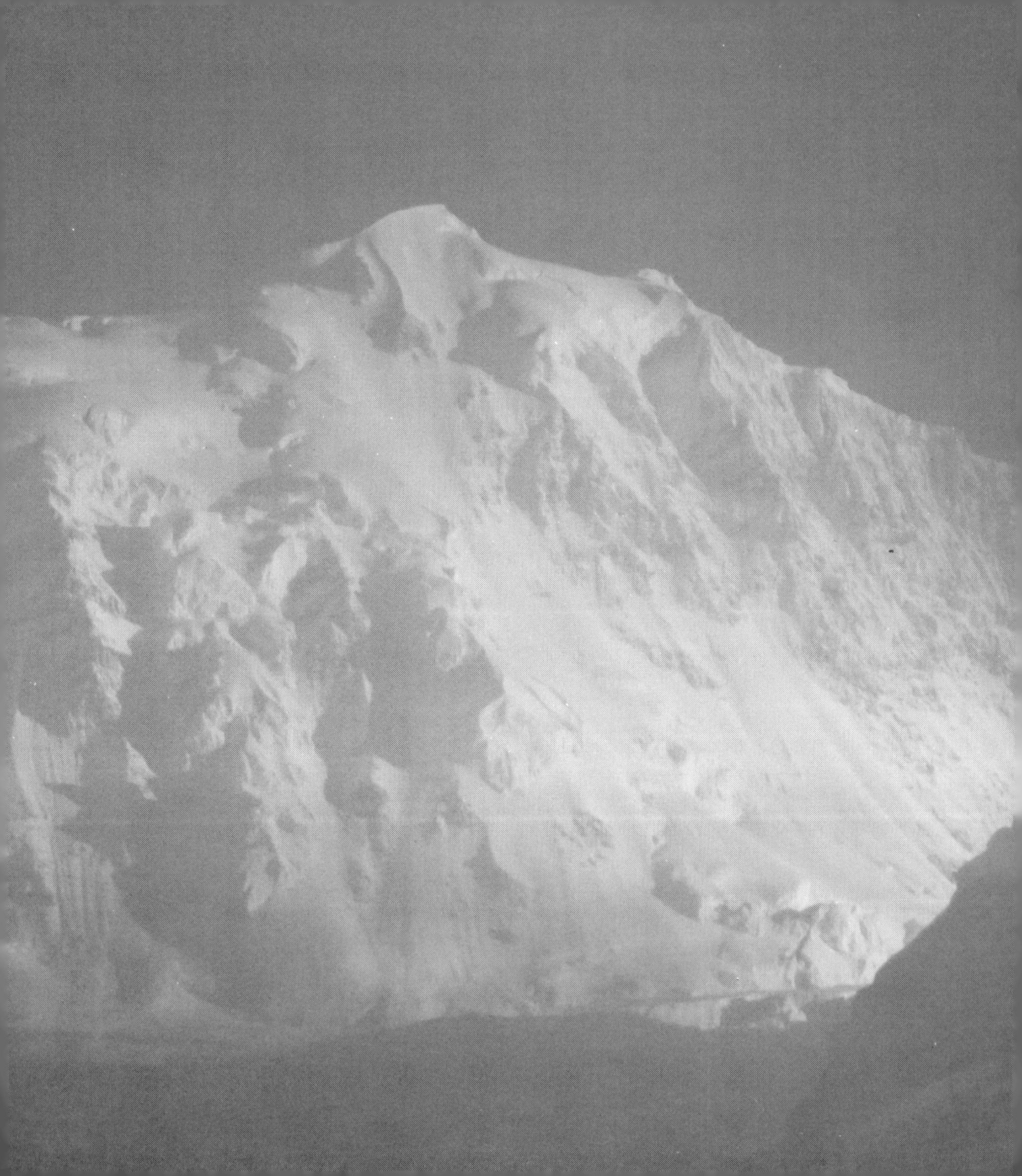

Ups and downs in life are very important, because a straight line, even in an ECG, means we are not alive.

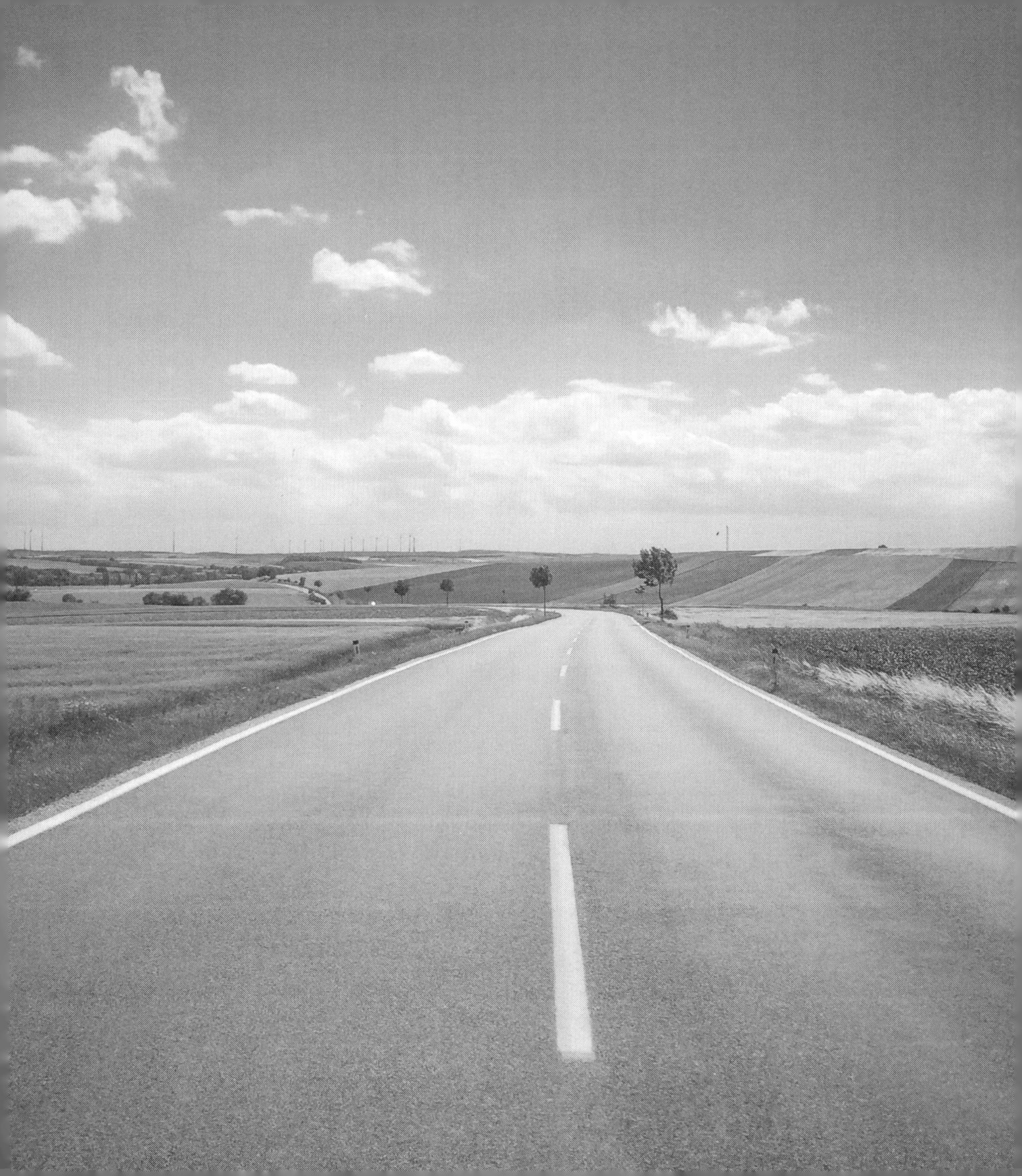

None can destroy iron but its own rust. Likewise, nothing can destroy a person but his own mindset.

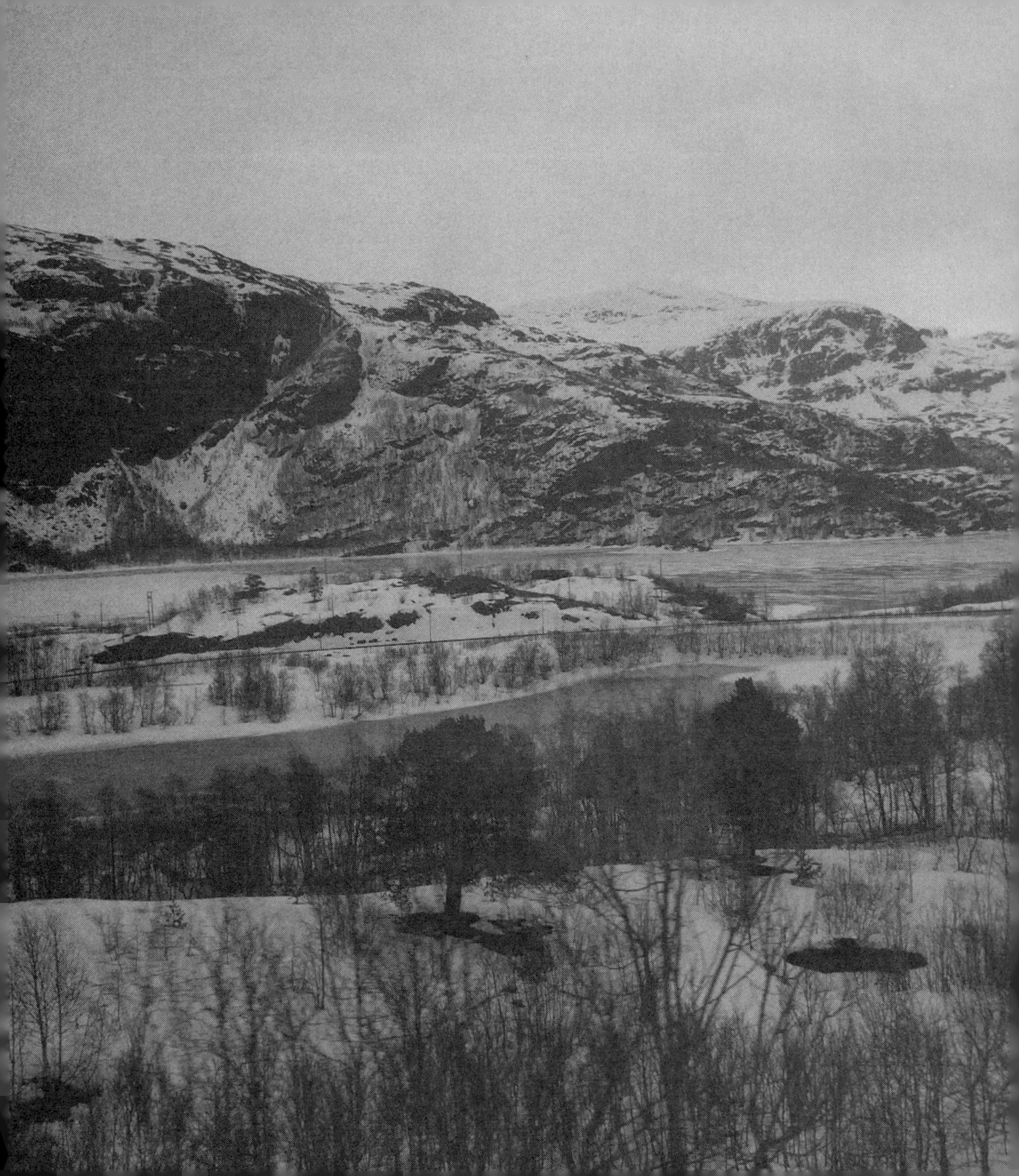

All of us do not have equal talent. Yet all of us can use an equal opportunity to develop our talent.

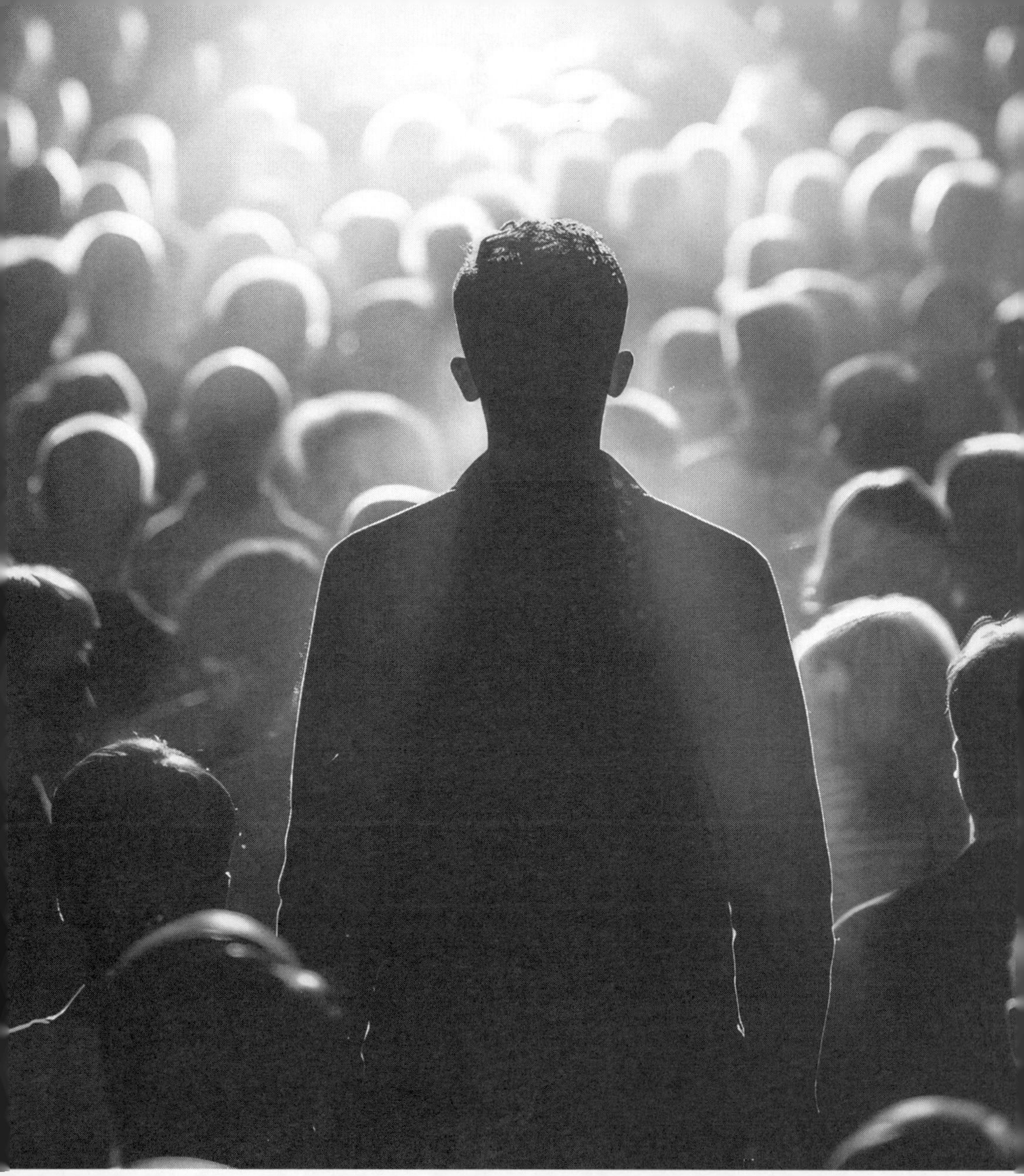

Leadership is about taking responsibility, not making excuses.

If there are challenges thrown across and those challenges are difficult, then some interesting, innovative solutions will come. If you don't have those challenges, then, I think, the tendency is to go on to say that whatever happens will happen in small deltas.

I would hope that as people who might take an elite position, would be considered amongst the elite in the country, you will always display humility in the manner in which you deal with your fellowmen, both in your company and in the country, and that you will continue to have passion in the areas in which you work.

(To college students.)

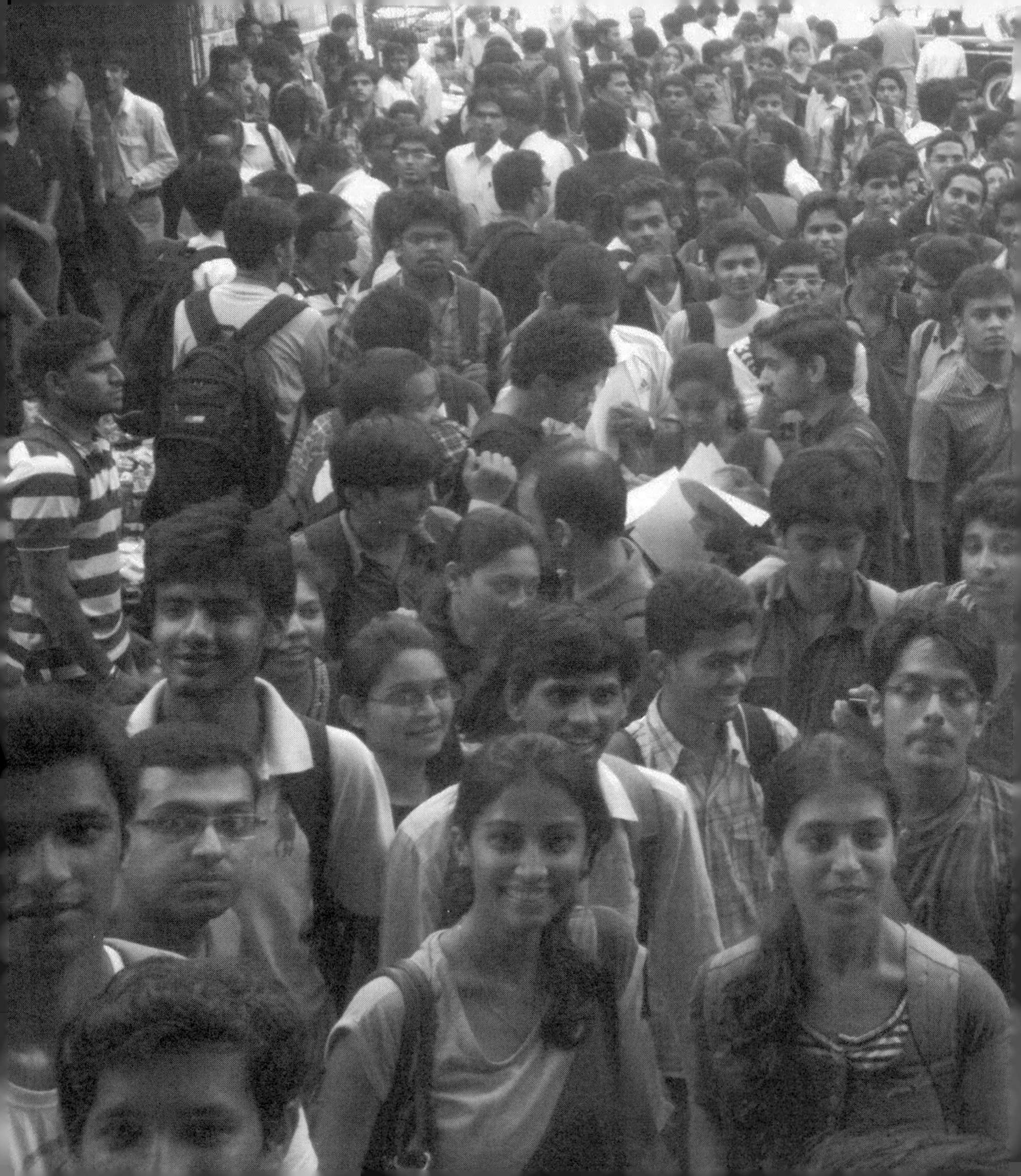

On many, many occasions you would have doubts on whether what you are pursuing is the right thing. But if you do believe in what you are trying to do and you pursue it and stay with it in a determined manner, I am quite sure you will succeed.

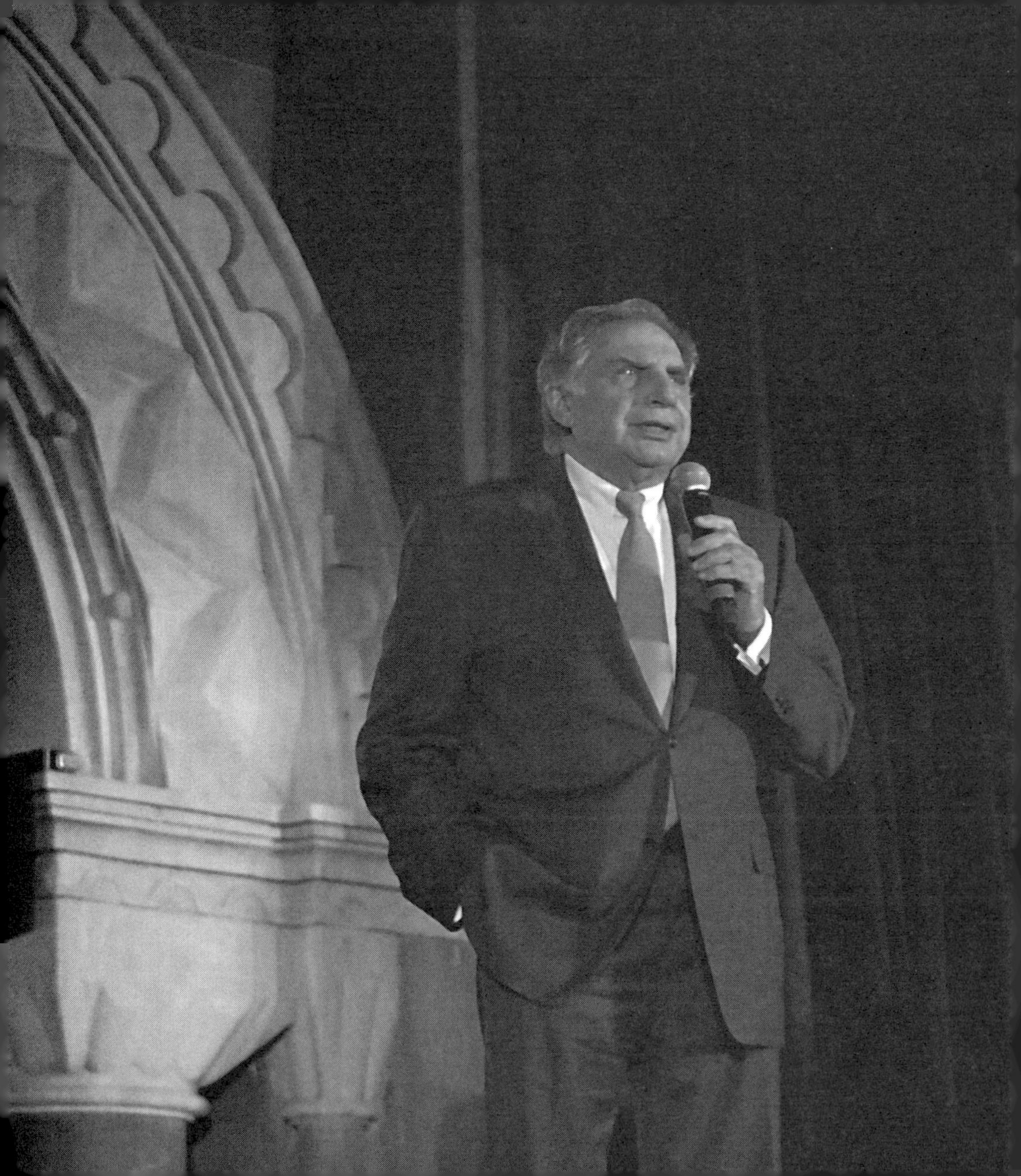

There are solutions for most problems. The barriers and roadblocks that we face are usually of our own making, and these can only be demolished by having the determination to find a solution — even if contrary to the conventional wisdom that prevails around us — by breaking tradition.

LOOKING WITHIN

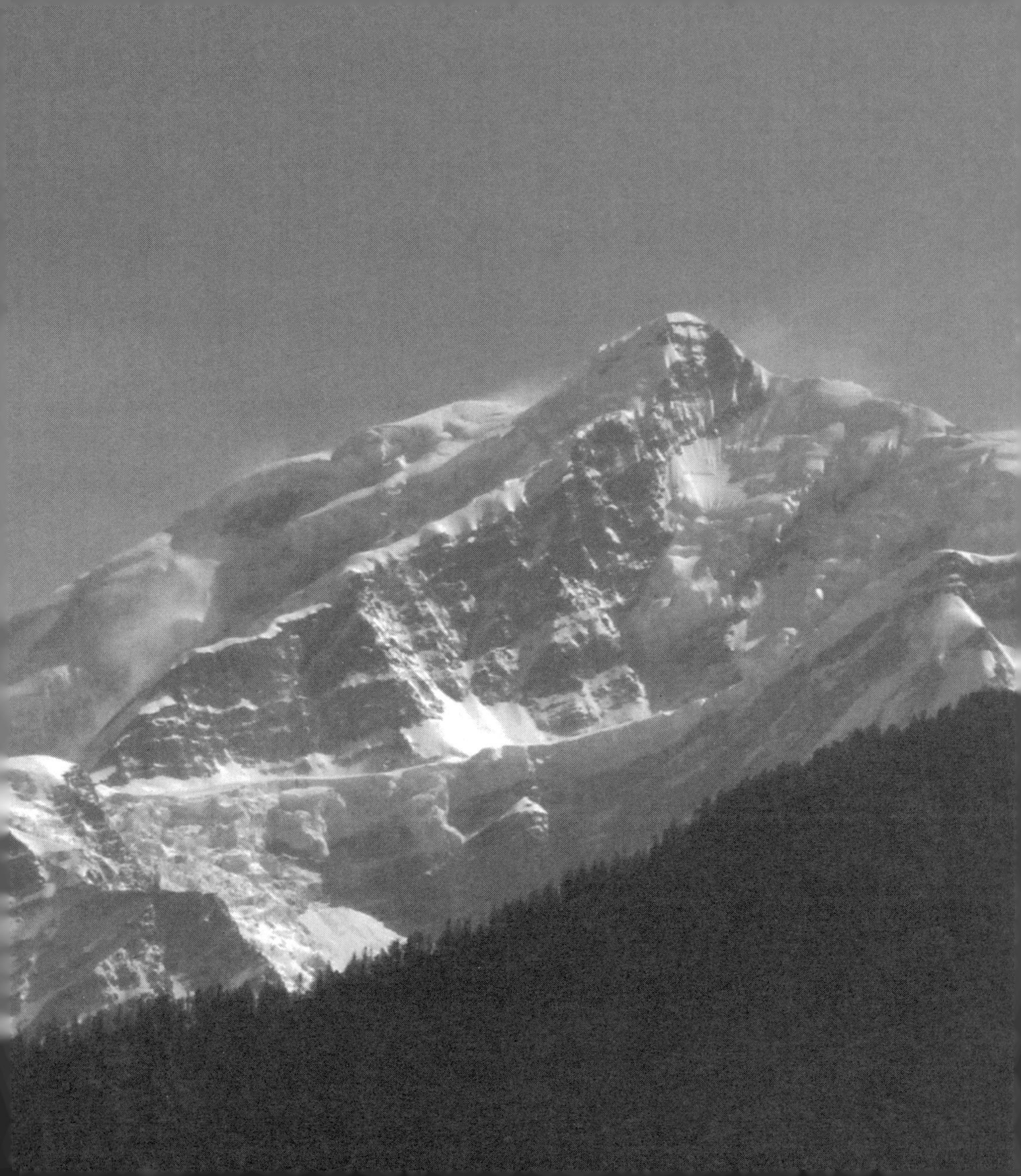

Be persistent and resilient in the face of challenges, for they are the building blocks of success.

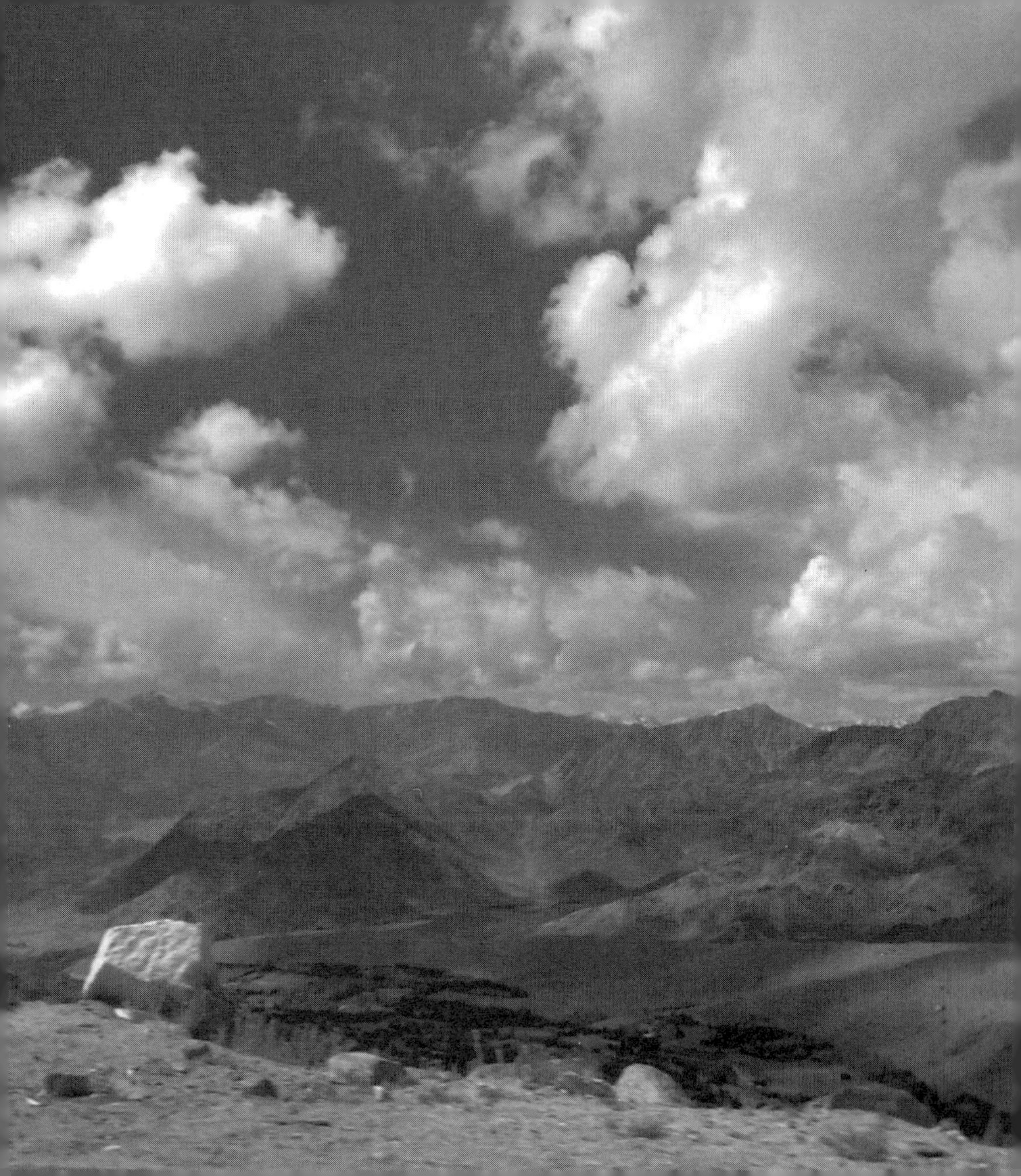

Power and wealth are not two of my main stakes.

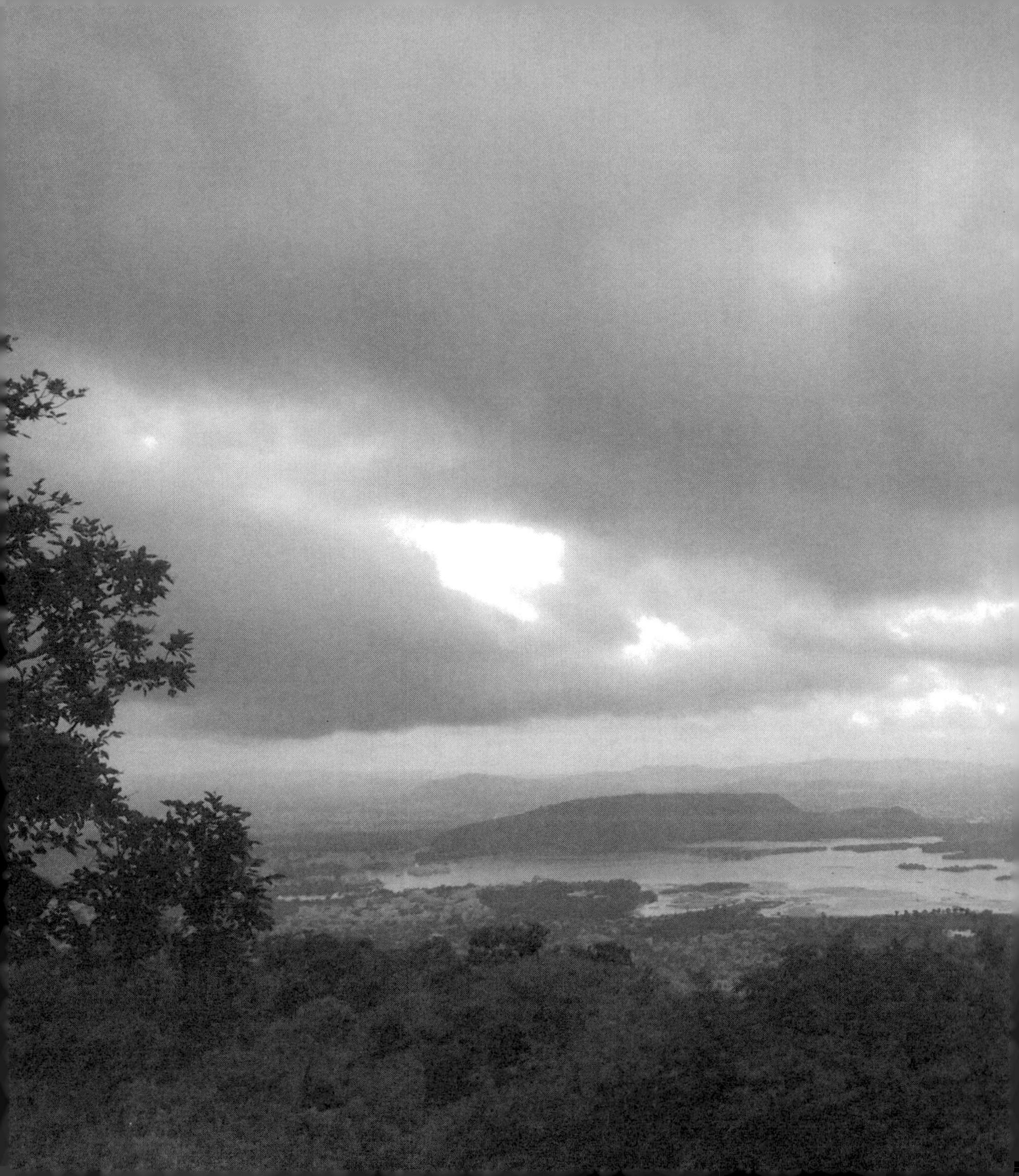

I don't believe in taking the right decision.
I take decisions and then make them right.

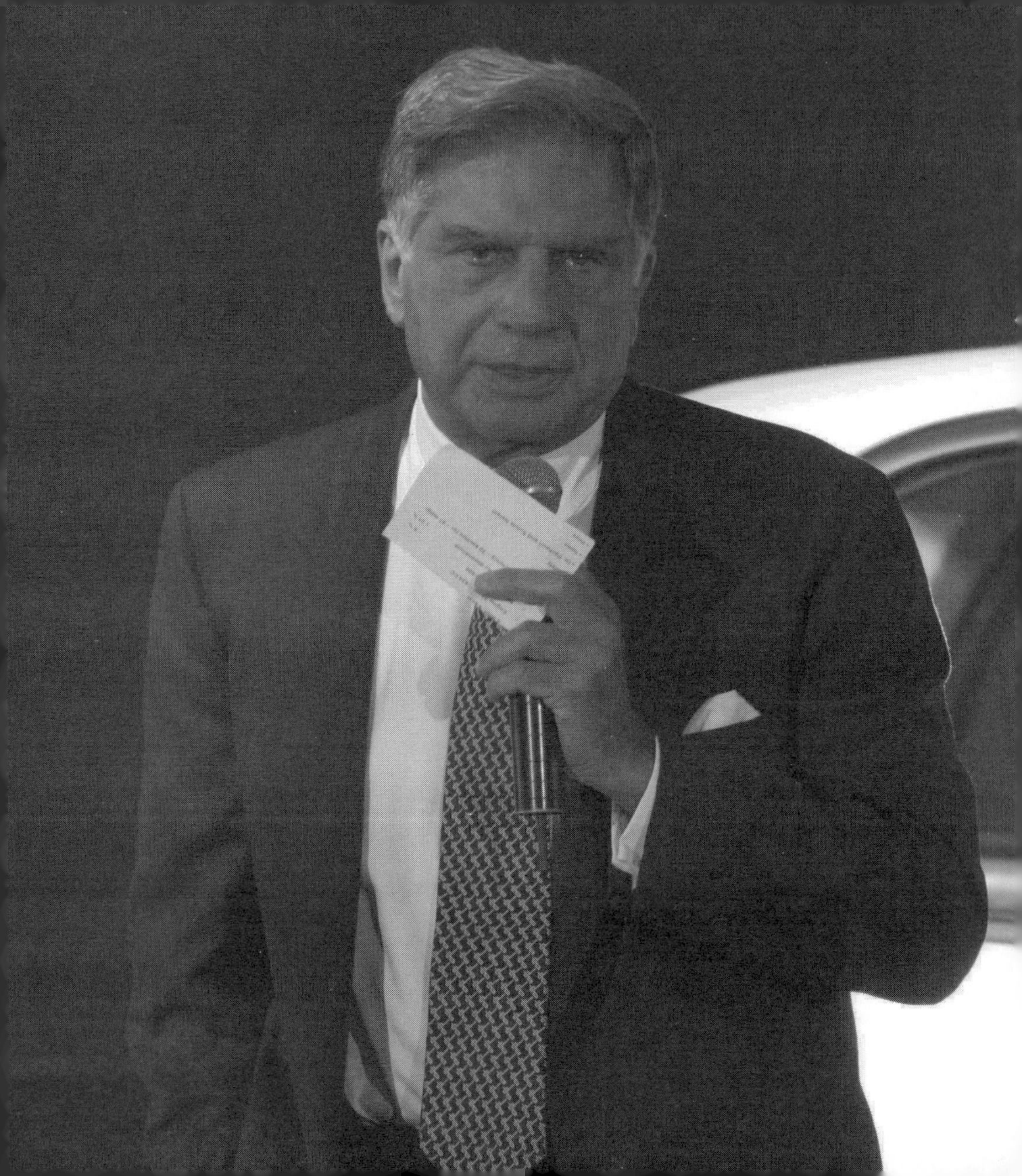

I believe I am a softer person today, maybe less decisive than I was when I took over, less idealistic, more pragmatic about what can be done and what cannot, and much more aware of the need to communicate.

(Eve of retirement.)

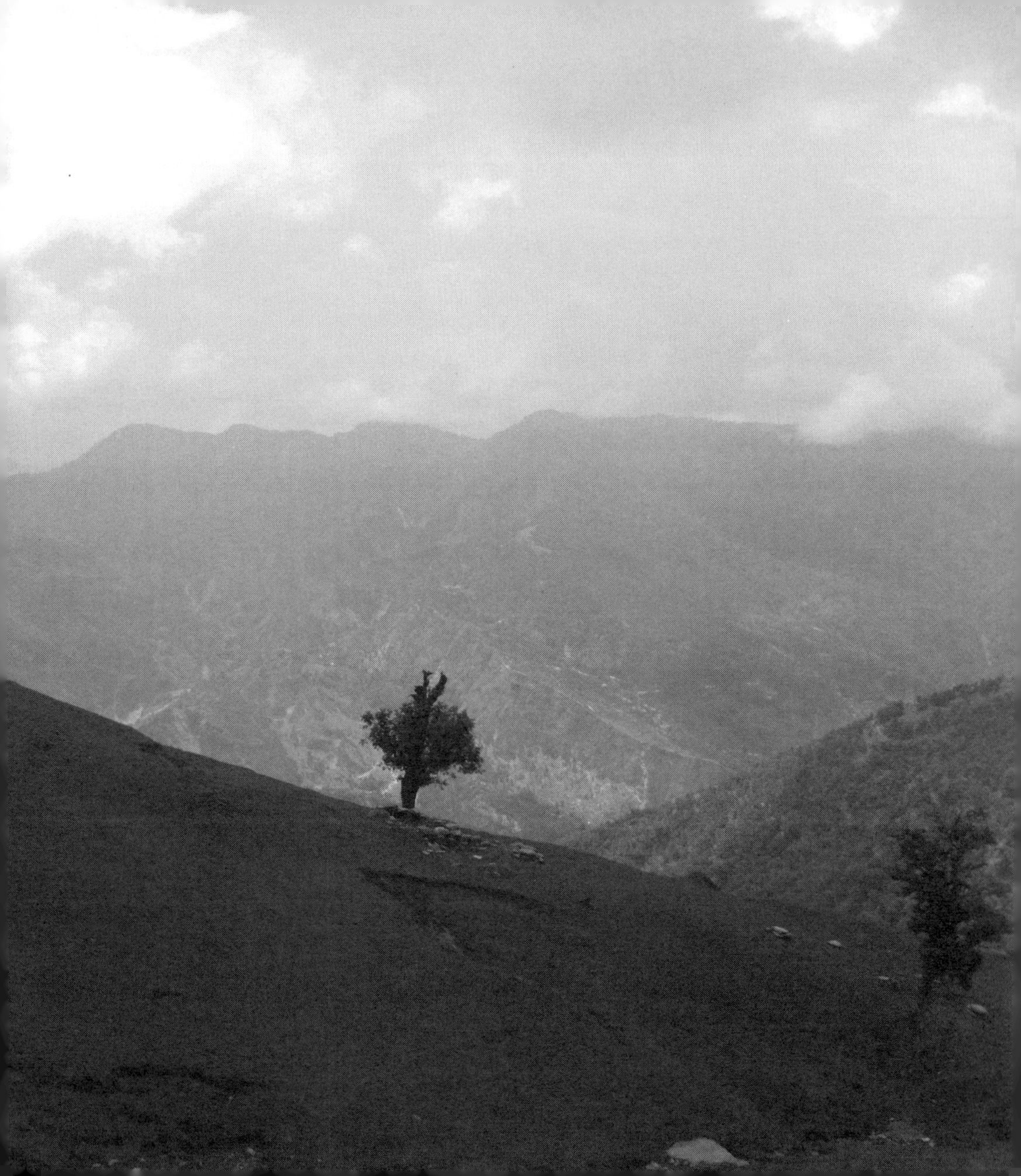

I am an introvert, kind of a private person, and I tried to remain that way. Some of the media glare I could not escape, so I faced up to it as part of the job. But in every other way, maybe to some extent to the detriment of the group and myself, I stayed away from the media unless I had to. I avoided being an easily accessible person and, as a consequence, the group has probably not had the visibility and the public relations positives that it should have garnered.

(Eve of retirement.)

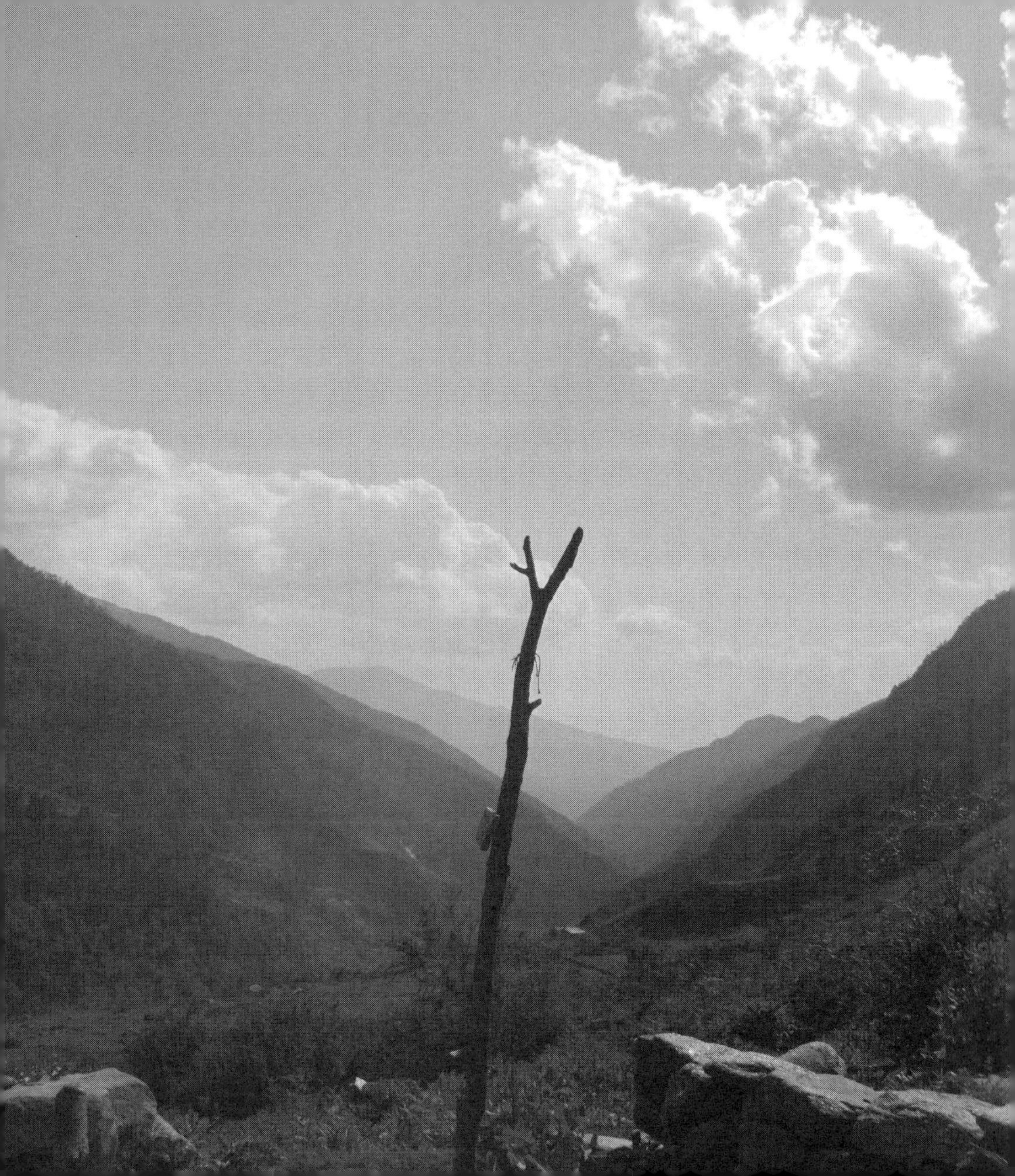

I came seriously close to getting married on four occasions and each time I backed off in fear, or for some reason or the other.

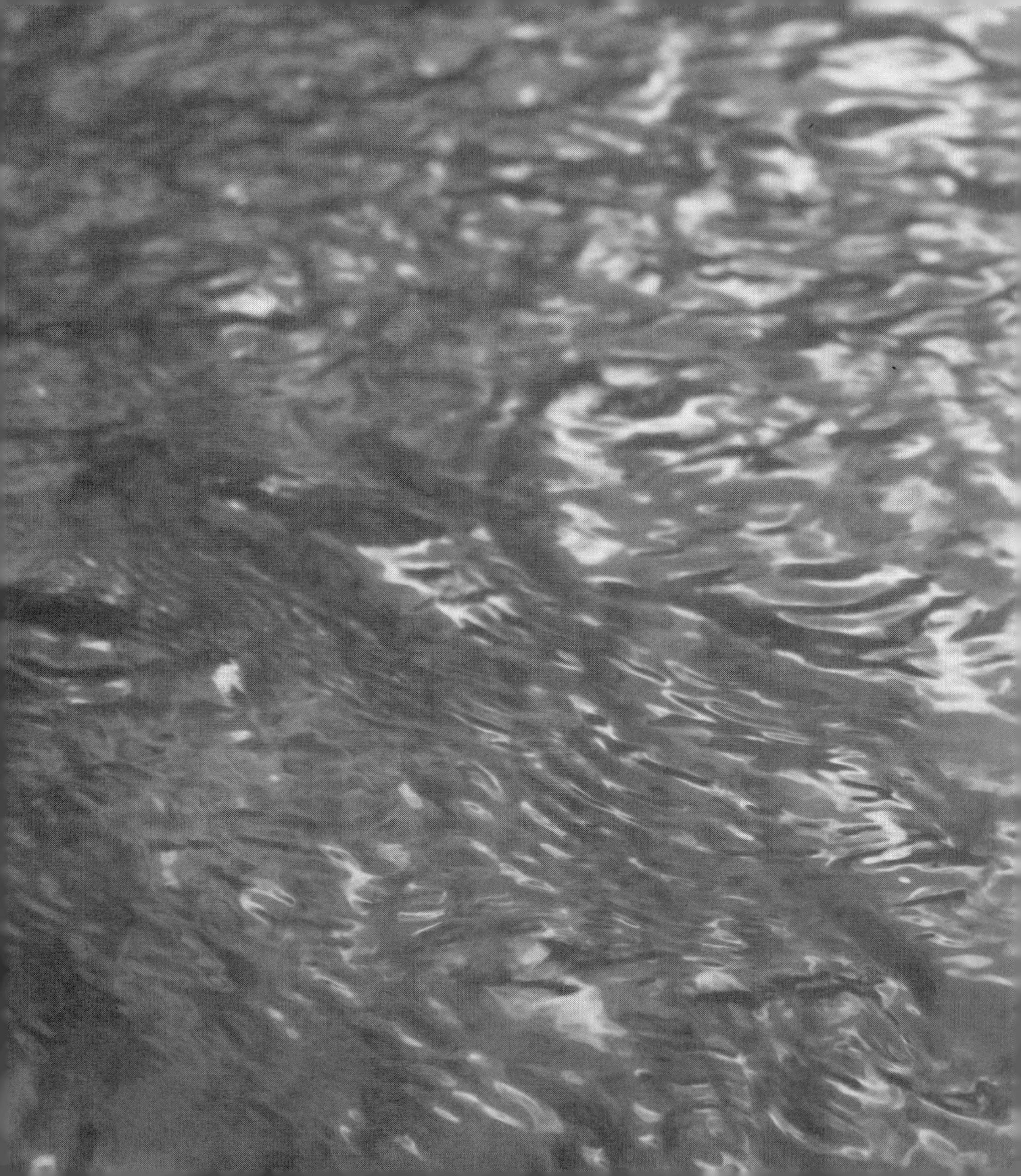

I am, unfortunately, a person who has often said: 'You put a gun to my head and pull the trigger or take the gun away; I won't move my head.'

(October 2008 while announcing the decision to shift the Nano project out of West Bengal.)

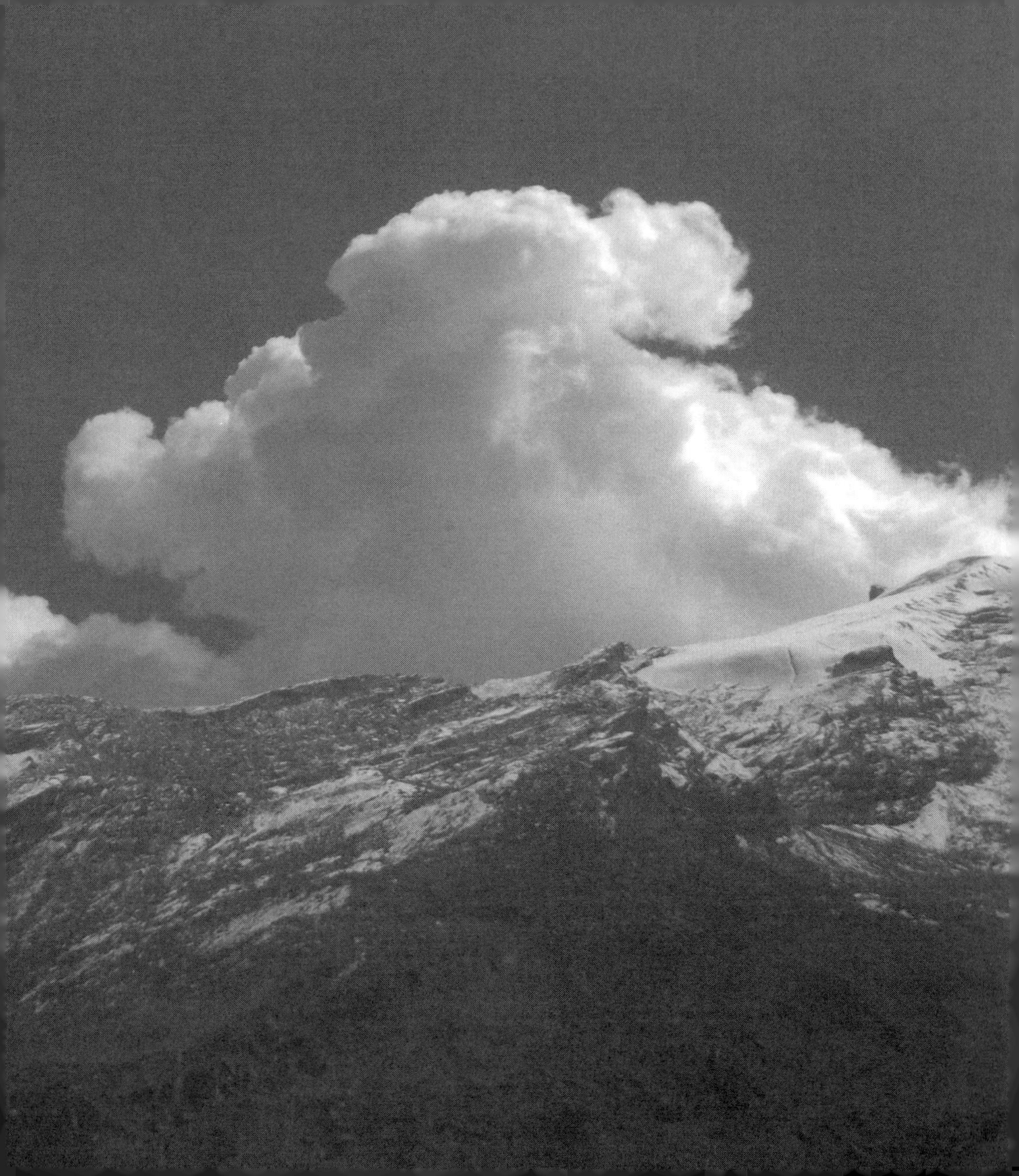

I seek perfection and this has been a source of motivation for me, as also frustration.

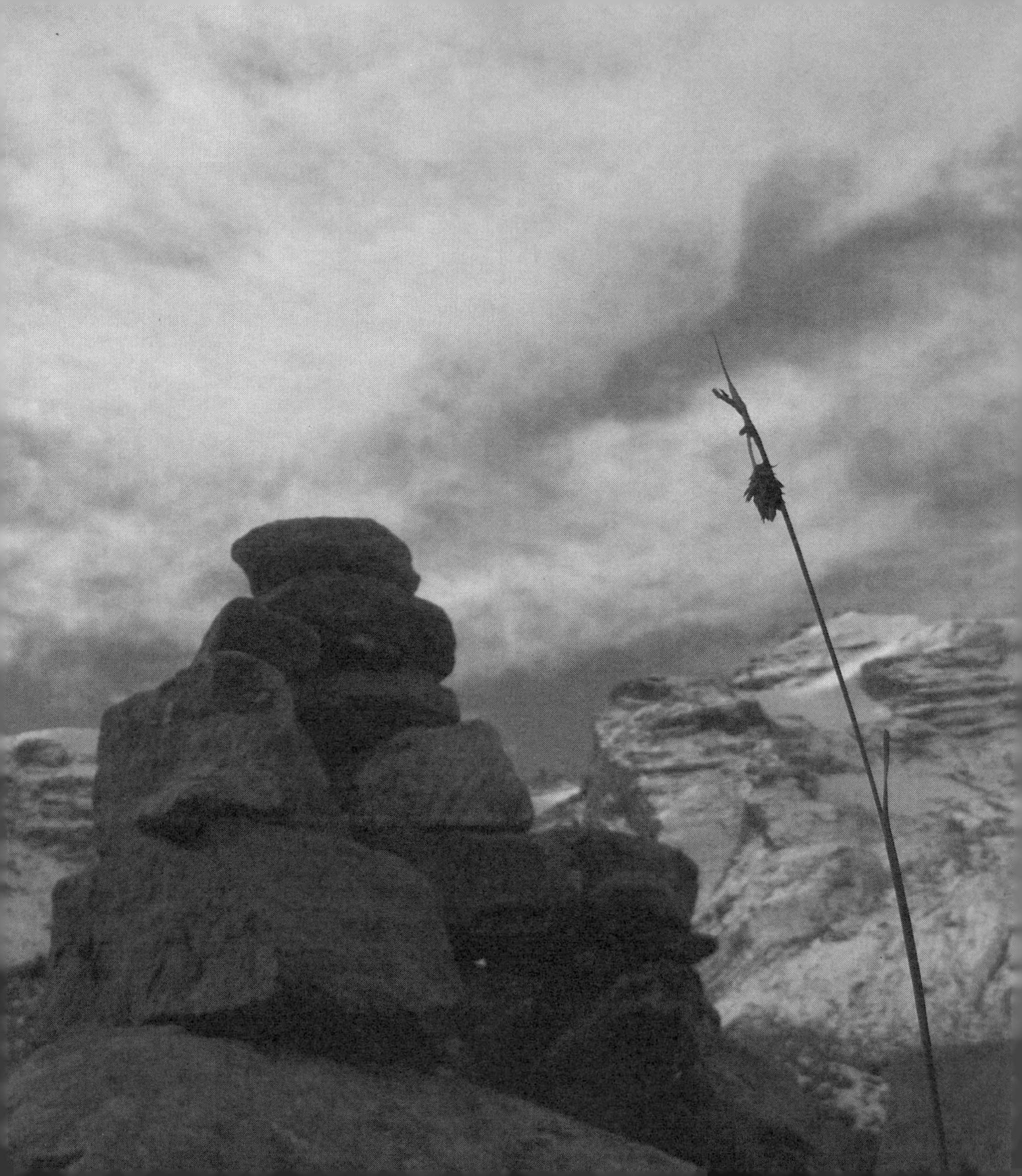

I admire people who are successful. But if that success has been achieved through too much ruthlessness, then I may admire that person, but I can't respect him.

I enjoy thinking about impossible things, and how I can perhaps actually make them possible.

LIFE

AFTER

RETIREMENT

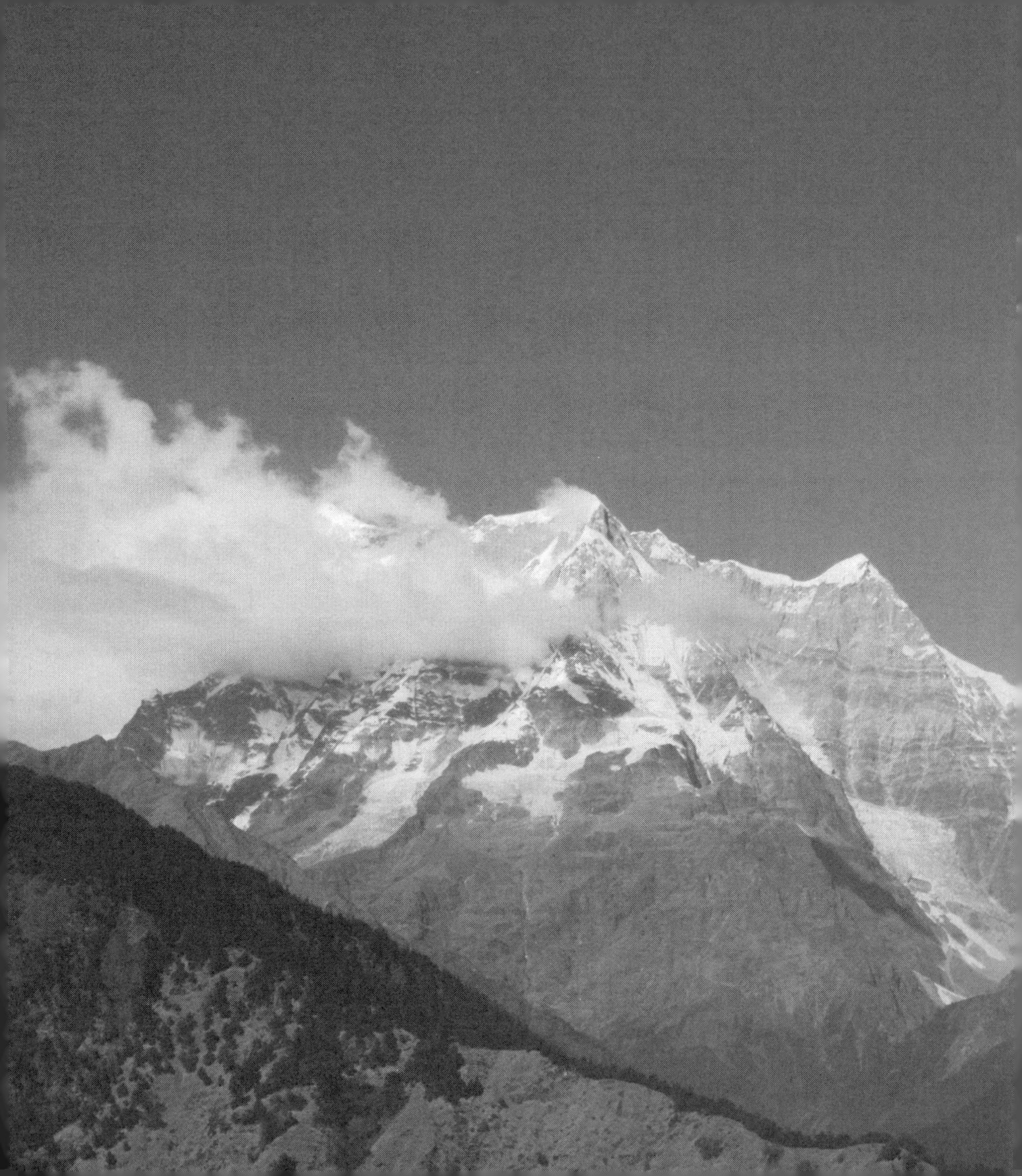

There has been more time to be at home, play with my dogs. There are things like music and painting that I used to be involved in. We always miss something that we did at one time and haven't had the chance to do since, and those kinds of things I probably want to try to get back to.

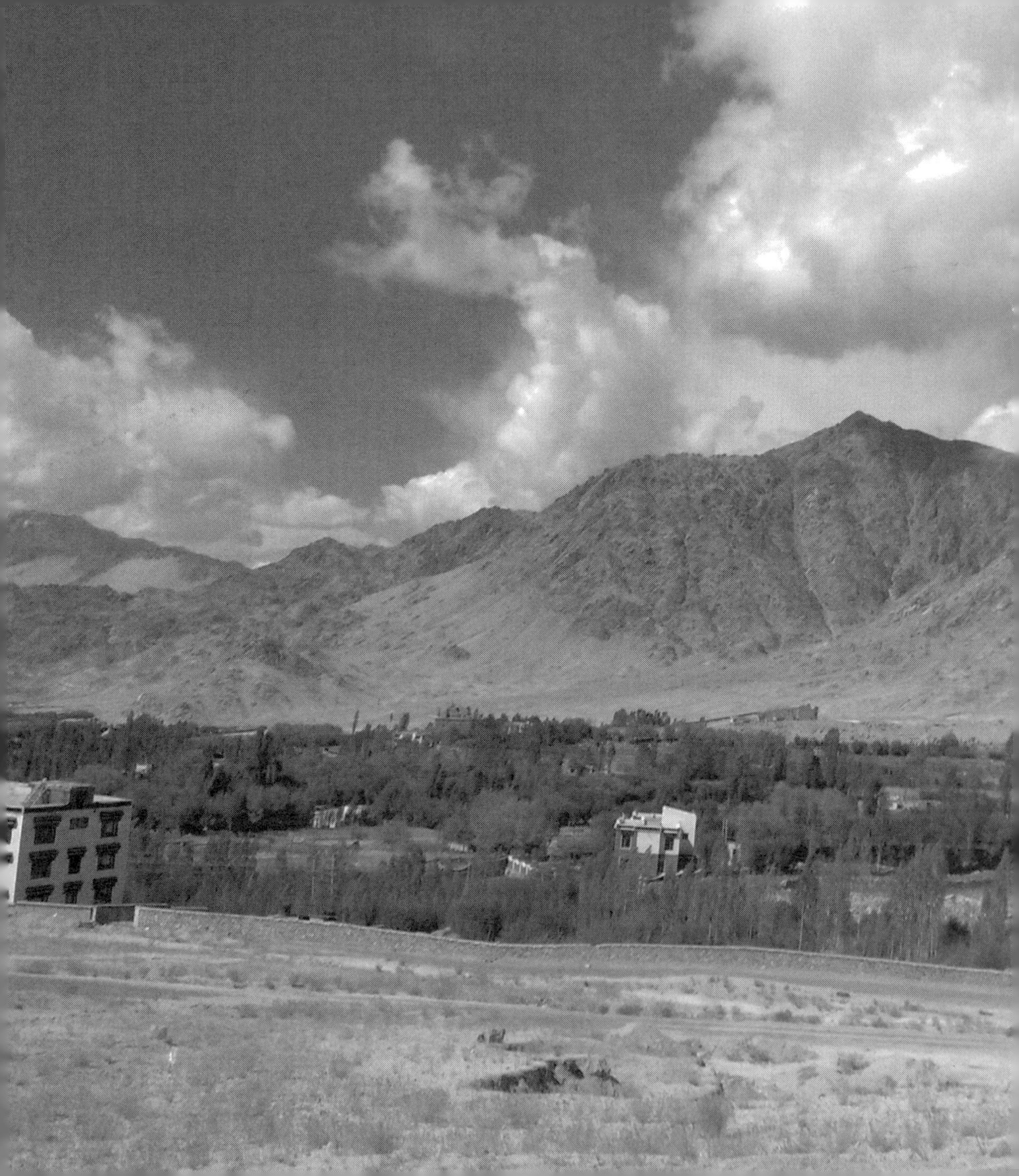

If I were a private citizen I would still be interested in establishing a world-class veterinary hospital. It would be in India and in Mumbai, specifically and selfishly, if I may add. Anybody who is an animal lover can see the complete void and lack of investment in facilities for the care of animals. You have to painfully watch if your pet is afflicted one way or another, without the necessary medical facilities or the expertise at hand to deal with the case. I believe all of us who have pets have experienced this.

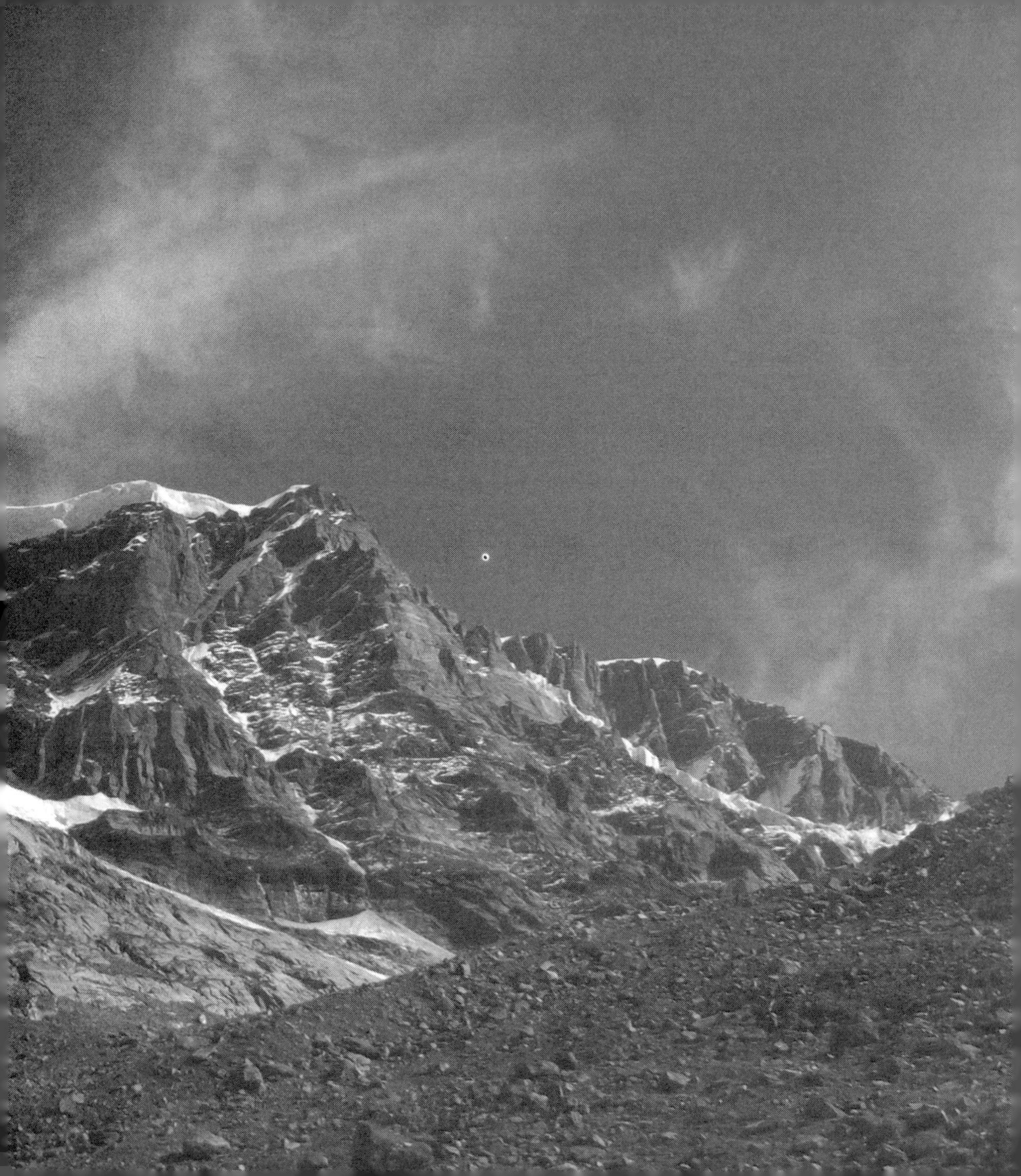

My most visible goal is to do something in nutrition for children in India and for pregnant mothers. That would change the mental and physical health of our population in years to come.

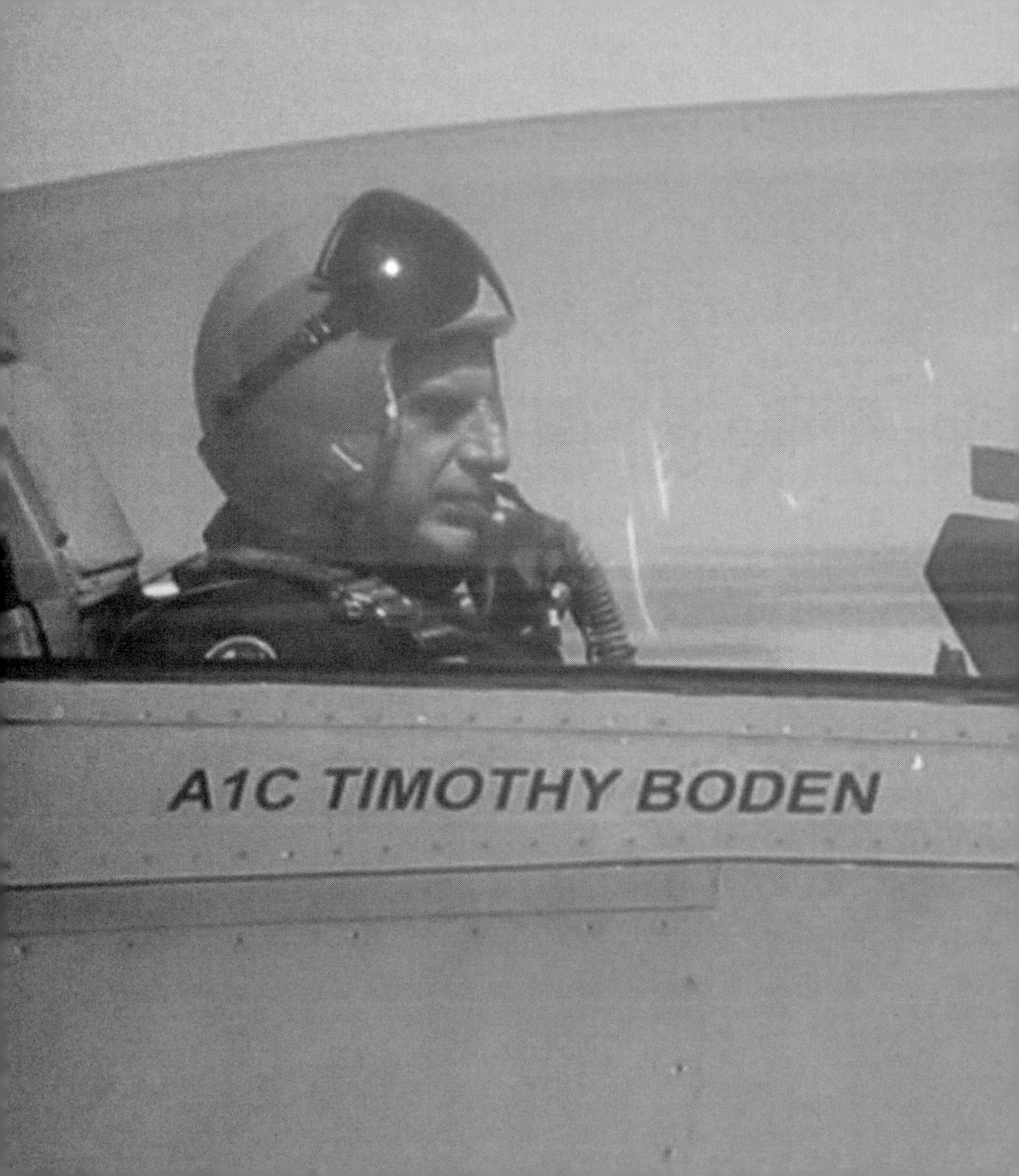
A1C TIMOTHY BODEN

Flying I continue to be involved with. I love flying and I hope to keep doing it so long as I can pass my medicals and stay proficient.

I do not know what the future holds,
but I do know that I'm going to be positively surprised.

'The gateways to wisdom and knowledge are always open.'

Louise Hay